T0226826

Antimicrobial Stewardship

Editor

CHESTON B. CUNHA

MEDICAL CLINICS OF NORTH AMERICA

www.medical.theclinics.com

Consulting Editor
BIMAL H. ASHAR

September 2018 • Volume 102 • Number 5

ELSEVIER

1600 John F. Kennedy Boulevard • Suite 1800 • Philadelphia, Pennsylvania, 19103-2899

http://www.theclinics.com

MEDICAL CLINICS OF NORTH AMERICA Volume 102, Number 5
September 2018 ISSN 0025-7125, ISBN-13: 978-0-323-61378-1

Editor: Jessica McCool
Developmental Editor: Kristen Helm

Medical Clinics of North America (ISSN 0025-7125) is published bimonthly by Elsevier Inc., 360 Park Avenue South, New York, NY 10010-1710. Months of publication are January, March, May, July, September, and November. Business and editorial offices: 1600 John F. Kennedy Boulevard, Suite 1800, Philadelphia, PA 19103-2899. Periodicals postage paid at New York, NY, and additional mailing offices. Subscription prices are USD $273.00 per year (US individuals), $574.00 per year (US institutions), $100.00 per year (US Students), $336.00 per year (Canadian individuals), $746.00 per year (Canadian institutions), $200.00 per year (Canadian and foreign students), $402.00 per year (foreign individuals), and $746.00 per year (foreign institutions). To receive student/resident rate, orders must be accompanied by name of affiliated institution, date of term, and the signature of program/residency coordinator on institution letterhead. Orders will be billed at individual rate until proof of status is received. Foreign air speed delivery is included in all Clinics' subscription prices. All prices are subject to change without notice. **POSTMASTER:** Send address changes to *Medical Clinics of North America*, Elsevier Health Sciences Division, Subscription Customer Service, 3251 Riverport Lane, Maryland Heights, MO 63043. **Customer Service: Telephone: 1-800-654-2452** (U.S. and Canada); **1-314-447-8871** (outside U.S. and Canada). **Fax: 314-447-8029. E-mail: journalscustomerserviceusa@elsevier.com** (for print support); **journalsonlinesupport-usa@elsevier.com** (for online support).

Reprints. For copies of 100 or more of articles in this publication, please contact the Commercial Reprints Department, Elsevier Inc., 360 Park Avenue South, New York, NY 10010-1710. Tel.: 212-633-3874; Fax: 212-633-3820; E-mail: reprints@elsevier.com.

Medical Clinics of North America is also published in Spanish by McGraw-Hill Interamericana Editores S. A., P.O. Box 5-237, 06500 Mexico, D.F., Mexico.

Medical Clinics of North America is covered in *MEDLINE/PubMed (Index Medicus), Current Contents, ASCA, Excerpta Medica, Science Citation Index,* and *ISI/BIOMED.*

PROGRAM OBJECTIVE
The goal of the *Medical Clinics of North America* is to keep practicing physicians up to date with current clinical practice by providing timely articles reviewing the state of the art in patient care.

TARGET AUDIENCE
All practicing physicians and other healthcare professionals.

LEARNING OBJECTIVES
Upon completion of this activity, participants will be able to:
1. Review current and future opportunities for rapid diagnostics in antimicrobial stewardship.
2. Discuss the roles of education, hospital epidemiologist, pharmacist, clinical microbiology laboratory and technology in antimicrobial stewardship.
3. Recognize pharmacoeconomic aspects of antibiotic stewardship programs.

ACCREDITATION
The Elsevier Office of Continuing Medical Education (EOCME) is accredited by the Accreditation Council for Continuing Medical Education (ACCME) to provide continuing medical education for physicians.

The EOCME designates this enduring material for a maximum of 15 *AMA PRA Category 1 Credit*(s)™. Physicians should claim only the credit commensurate with the extent of their participation in the activity.

All other healthcare professionals requesting continuing education credit for this enduring material will be issued a certificate of participation.

DISCLOSURE OF CONFLICTS OF INTEREST
The EOCME assesses conflict of interest with its instructors, faculty, planners, and other individuals who are in a position to control the content of CME activities. All relevant conflicts of interest that are identified are thoroughly vetted by EOCME for fair balance, scientific objectivity, and patient care recommendations. EOCME is committed to providing its learners with CME activities that promote improvements or quality in healthcare and not a specific proprietary business or a commercial interest.

The planning committee, staff, authors and editors listed below have identified no financial relationships or relationships to products or devices they or their spouse/life partner have with commercial interest related to the content of this CME activity:
Salma Abbas, MBBS; Bimal H. Ashar, MD, MBA, FACP; Emilio Bouza, MD, PhD; Derek N. Bremmer, PharmD; Amy L. Brotherton, PharmD; Almudena Burillo, MD, PhD; Cheston B. Cunha, MD, FACP; Yi Guo, PharmD; Inge C. Gyssens, MD, PhD; Alison Kemp; Jessica McCool; Matthew A. Moffa, DO; Jacob Morton, PharmD, MBA, BCPS; Patricia Muñoz, MD, PhD; Priya Nori, MD; Steven M. Opal, MD; Belinda Ostrowsky, MD, MPH, FIDSA, FSHEA; Diane M. Parente, PharmD; Edward Joel Septimus, MD; Emily S. Spivak, MD, MHS; Michael P. Stevens, MD, MPH; Jeyanthi Surendrakumar; Tristan T. Timbrook, PharmD, MBA; Tamara L. Trienski, PharmD; John J. Veillette, PharmD; Todd J. Vento, MD, MPH; Thomas L. Walsh, MD.

The planning committee, staff, authors and editors listed below have identified financial relationships or relationships to products or devices they or their spouse/life partner have with commercial interest related to the content of this CME activity:
Whitney R. Buckel, PharmD: is a consultant/advisor for Merck & Co, Inc
Kimberly E. Hanson, MD, MHS: receives research support from BioFire Diagnostics
Louis B. Rice, MD: is a consultant/advisor for Macrolide Pharmaceuticals and Zavante Therapeutics, Inc.
Edward A. Stenehjem, MD, MSc: receives research support from Pfizer Inc. and Allergan
Tristan T. Timbrook, PharmD, MBA: is a speaker and a consultant/advisor for BioFire Diagnostics, GenMark Diagnostics, Inc., and F. Hoffmann-La Roche Ltd

UNAPPROVED/OFF-LABEL USE DISCLOSURE
The EOCME requires CME faculty to disclose to the participants:
1. When products or procedures being discussed are off-label, unlabelled, experimental, and/or investigational (not US Food and Drug Administration [FDA] approved); and
2. Any limitations on the information presented, such as data that are preliminary or that represent ongoing research, interim analyses, and/or unsupported opinions. Faculty may discuss information about pharmaceutical agents that is outside of FDA-approved labelling. This information is intended solely for CME and is not intended to promote off-label use of these medications. If you have any questions, contact the medical affairs department of the manufacturer for the most recent prescribing information.

TO ENROLL

To enroll in the *Medical Clinics of North America* Continuing Medical Education program, call customer service at 1-800-654-2452 or sign up online at http://www.theclinics.com/home/cme. The CME program is available to subscribers for an additional annual fee of USD $300.90.

METHOD OF PARTICIPATION

In order to claim credit, participants must complete the following:

1. Complete enrolment as indicated above.
2. Read the activity.
3. Complete the CME Test and Evaluation. Participants must achieve a score of 70% on the test. All CME Tests and Evaluations must be completed online.

CME INQUIRIES/SPECIAL NEEDS

For all CME inquiries or special needs, please contact elsevierCME@elsevier.com.

MEDICAL CLINICS OF NORTH AMERICA

FORTHCOMING ISSUES

November 2018
Otolaryngology
C. Matthew Stewart, *Editor*

January 2019
Gastroenterology for the Internist
Kerry B. Dunbar, *Editor*

March 2019
Neurology for the Non-Neurologist
Tracey A. Milligan, *Editor*

RECENT ISSUES

July 2018
Substance Use and Addiction Medicine
Jeffrey H. Samet, Patrick G. O'Connor, and
Michael D. Stein, *Editors*

May 2018
Clinical Examination
Brian T. Garibaldi, *Editor*

March 2018
Urology
Robert E. Brannigan, *Editor*

ISSUE OF RELATED INTEREST

Infectious Disease Clinics of North America, December 2017 (Vol. 31, No. 4)
Infections in Older Adults
Robin L.P. Jump and David H. Canaday, *Editors*
Available at: http://www.id.theclinics.com/

Contributors

CONSULTING EDITOR

BIMAL H. ASHAR, MD, MBA, FACP
Associate Professor of Medicine, Division of General Internal Medicine, Johns Hopkins School of Medicine, Baltimore, Maryland, USA

EDITOR

CHESTON B. CUNHA, MD, FACP
Assistant Professor of Medicine, The Warren Alpert Medical School of Brown University, Medical Director, Antibiotic Stewardship Program (Rhode Island Hospital and The Miriam Hospital), Division of Infectious Disease, Rhode Island Hospital, Providence, Rhode Island, USA

AUTHORS

SALMA ABBAS, MBBS
Division of Infectious Diseases, Virginia Commonwealth University, Richmond, Virginia, USA

EMILIO BOUZA, MD, PhD
Clinical Professor Emeritus, Medicine Department, School of Medicine, Universidad Complutense de Madrid (UCM), Instituto de Investigación Sanitaria Gregorio Marañón, Department of Clinical Microbiology and Infectious Diseases, Hospital General Universitario Gregorio Marañón, CIBER de Enfermedades Respiratorias (CIBERES CB06/06/0058), Madrid, Spain

DEREK N. BREMMER, PharmD
Department of Pharmacy, Allegheny General Hospital, Allegheny Health Network, Pittsburgh, Pennsylvania, USA

AMY L. BROTHERTON, PharmD
Clinical Pharmacist Specialist, Infectious Diseases, Department of Pharmacy, The Miriam Hospital, Providence, Rhode Island, USA

WHITNEY R. BUCKEL, PharmD
Intermountain Healthcare Pharmacy Services, Taylorsville, Utah, USA

ALMUDENA BURILLO, MD, PhD
Medicine Department, School of Medicine, Universidad Complutense de Madrid (UCM), Instituto de Investigación Sanitaria Gregorio Marañón, Department of Clinical Microbiology and Infectious Diseases, Hospital General Universitario Gregorio Marañón, Madrid, Spain

CHESTON B. CUNHA, MD, FACP
Assistant Professor of Medicine, The Warren Alpert Medical School of Brown University, Medical Director, Antibiotic Stewardship Program (Rhode Island Hospital and The Miriam Hospital), Division of Infectious Disease, Rhode Island Hospital, Providence, Rhode Island, USA

YI GUO, PharmD
Department of Pharmacy, Antimicrobial Stewardship Program, Montefiore Health System, Albert Einstein College of Medicine, Bronx, New York, USA

INGE C. GYSSENS, MD, PhD
Professor, Department of Medicine, Radboud University Medical Center, Nijmegen, The Netherlands; Faculty of Medicine, Research Group of Immunology and Biochemistry, Hasselt University, Hasselt, Belgium

KIMBERLY E. HANSON, MD, MHS
Institute for Clinical and Experimental Pathology, ARUP Laboratories, Departments of Medicine and Pathology, The University of Utah, Salt Lake City, Utah, USA

MATTHEW A. MOFFA, DO
Division of Infectious Diseases, Allegheny General Hospital, Allegheny Health Network, Pittsburgh, Pennsylvania, USA

JACOB MORTON, PharmD, MBA, BCPS
Clinical Pharmacy Coordinator, Infectious Diseases, Department of Pharmacy, Saint Vincent Hospital, Worcester, Massachusetts, USA

PATRICIA MUÑOZ, MD, PhD
Medicine Department, School of Medicine, Universidad Complutense de Madrid (UCM), Instituto de Investigación Sanitaria Gregorio Marañón, CIBER de Enfermedades Respiratorias (CIBERES CB06/06/0058), Department of Clinical Microbiology and Infectious Diseases, Hospital General Universitario Gregorio Marañón, Madrid, Spain

PRIYA NORI, MD
Assistant Professor of Clinical Medicine, Division of Infectious Diseases, Antimicrobial Stewardship Program, Montefiore Health System, Albert Einstein College of Medicine, Bronx, New York, USA

STEVEN M. OPAL, MD
Division of Infectious Disease, Rhode Island Hospital, The Miriam Hospital, The Warren Alpert Medical School of Brown University, Providence, Rhode Island, USA

BELINDA OSTROWSKY, MD, MPH, FIDSA, FSHEA
Associate Professor of Clinical Medicine, Division of Infectious Diseases, Antimicrobial Stewardship Program, Montefiore Health System, Albert Einstein College of Medicine, Bronx, New York, USA

DIANE M. PARENTE, PharmD
Clinical Pharmacist Specialist, Infectious Diseases and Antimicrobial Stewardship, Department of Pharmacy, The Miriam Hospital, Providence, Rhode Island, USA

LOUIS B. RICE, MD
Department of Medicine, The Warren Alpert Medical School of Brown University, Rhode Island Hospital, Providence, Rhode Island, USA

EDWARD JOEL SEPTIMUS, MD
Texas A&M College of Medicine, Houston, Texas, USA

EMILY S. SPIVAK, MD, MHS
Department of Medicine, The University of Utah, Salt Lake City, Utah, USA

EDWARD STENEHJEM, MD, MSc
Intermountain Healthcare and TeleHealth Service, Murray, Utah, USA

MICHAEL P. STEVENS, MD, MPH
Division of Infectious Diseases, Virginia Commonwealth University, Richmond, Virginia, USA

TRISTAN T. TIMBROOK, PharmD, MBA
Department of Pharmacy, The University of Utah, Salt Lake City, Utah, USA

TAMARA L. TRIENSKI, PharmD
Department of Pharmacy, Allegheny General Hospital, Allegheny Health Network, Pittsburgh, Pennsylvania, USA

JOHN J. VEILLETTE, PharmD
Division of Infectious Diseases and Epidemiology, Intermountain Infectious Diseases TeleHealth Service, Murray, Utah, USA

TODD J. VENTO, MD, MPH
Intermountain Infectious Diseases TeleHealth Service, Murray, Utah, USA

THOMAS L. WALSH, MD
Division of Infectious Diseases, Allegheny General Hospital, Allegheny Health Network, Pittsburgh, Pennsylvania, USA

Contents

> Antimicrobial stewardship involves optimizing antibiotic use while using
> cost-effective interventions to minimize antibiotic resistance and control
> *Clostridium difficile*. An effective hospital-wide antimicrobial stewardship
> program (ASP) should be led by an infectious disease (ID) physician. The
> ASP team needs full and ongoing financial support for the ASP from the hos-
> pital administration. The ID clinician leader should have special expertise in
> various aspects of antimicrobial therapy, that is, pharmacokinetics, resis-
> tance, pharmacoeconomics, and *C difficile*. The ASP ID team leader and
> ID-trained clinical pharmacist staff are responsible for customizing ASP in-
> terventions to the hospital's unique set of antibiotic use-related concerns.

> Antimicrobial stewardship programs aim to reduce costs, optimize thera-
> peutic outcomes, and reduce antimicrobial resistance. Reductions of anti-
> microbial resistance are the most elusive because emergence and spread
> of resistant bacteria involves antimicrobial selective pressure and lapses in
> infection control techniques. The relationship between antimicrobial usage
> and resistance is not always direct. The understanding of which techniques
> are most effective is limited because many studies are descriptive or qua-
> siexperimental. Recent meta-analyses or systematic reviews of steward-
> ship programs offer encouragement that some interventions reduce
> overall antimicrobial selective pressure and, where associated with infec-
> tion control interventions, affect resistance rates in individual institutions.

> Antimicrobial resistance (AR) is one of the most serious public health
> threats today, which has been accelerated by the overuse and misuse of

antimicrobials in humans and animals plus inadequate infection prevention. Numerous studies have shown a relationship between antimicrobial use and resistance. Antimicrobial stewardship (AS) programs have been shown to improve patient outcomes, reduce antimicrobial adverse events, and decrease AR. AS programs, when implemented alongside infection control measures, especially hand-hygiene interventions, were more effective than implementation of AS alone. Targeted coordination and prevention strategies are critical to stopping the spread of multidrug-resistant organisms.

Empiric therapy of the septic patient in the hospital is challenging. Antibiotic stewardship is concerned with optimizing antibiotic use and minimizing resistance. Clinicians should avoid overcovering and overtreating colonizing organisms in respiratory secretions and urinary catheters. Empiric therapy should take into account the prevalence of multidrug-resistant organisms in the hospital setting. The most effective resistance prevention strategy is to preferentially select a low resistance potential antibiotic, which should be administered in the highest possible dose without toxicity for the shortest duration to eliminate the infection.

Antimicrobial stewardship program (ASP) success and growth rely on recurring collaborations with partners within the health care system, such as administration, clinical services, infection prevention, pharmacy, the medical school, and microbiology. These collaborations present valuable opportunities for development of hospital policies, institutional guidelines, and educational curriculum. External opportunities for collaboration may be less frequent but equally valuable. These collaborations are facilitated by health system partnerships with national quality organizations, neighboring ASPs, and the Department of Health. All collaborations present novel opportunities for policy development, research initiatives, and expanding the regional ASP footprint.

The ability to treat infectious diseases with antimicrobials is an essential component of medical management. Antimicrobial therapy is based on the characteristics of the patient, drug, microorganisms causing the infection, and colonizing flora. Prudent antibiotic use is the only option to delay the emergence of resistance. Training in infectious diseases and knowledge of the principles of responsible antibiotic prescribing and uses must be improved. To change practice, health care professionals should be educated at all levels of their training.

Antibiotic stewardship programs (ASPs) play a crucial role in controlling the emergence of resistant organisms, reducing rates of *Clostridium difficile* infections and associated hospital length of stay, promoting judicious use of antibiotics, and minimizing associated adverse events. There is a significant overlap between the goals of infection control programs and ASPs, and both programs can benefit from a synergistic relationship. Hospital epidemiologists can support these programs by providing leadership support, sharing surveillance data, bridging gaps between ASPs and departments such as microbiology, integrating educational programs with ASPs, sharing outbreak alerts, and assisting with the development of treatment algorithms.

For adequate antimicrobial stewardship, microbiology needs to move from the laboratory to become physically and verbally amenable to the caregivers of an institution. Herein, the authors describe the contributions of their microbiology department to the antimicrobial stewardship program of a large teaching hospital as 10 main points ranging from the selection of patients deemed likely to benefit from a fast track approach, to their clinical samples, or the rapid reporting of results via a microbiology hotline, to rapid searches for pathogens and susceptibility testing. These points should serve as guidelines for similar programs designed to decrease the unnecessary use of antimicrobials.

Rapid diagnostic testing has improved clinical care of patients with infectious syndromes when combined with antimicrobial stewardship. The authors review the current data on antimicrobial stewardship and rapid diagnostic testing in bloodstream, respiratory tract, and gastrointestinal tract infections. Evidence for the potential benefit of rapid tests in bloodstream infections seems strong, respiratory tract infections mixed, and gastrointestinal tract infections still evolving. The authors also review future directions in rapid diagnostic testing and suggest areas of focus for antimicrobial stewardship efforts.

Antibiotic stewardship programs are needed in all health care facilities, regardless of size and location. Community hospitals that have fewer resources may have different priorities and require different strategies when defining antibiotic stewardship program components and implementing interventions. By following the Centers for Disease Control and Prevention Core Elements and using the strategies suggested in this article, readers should be able to design, develop, participate in, or improve antibiotic stewardship programs within community hospitals.

The goals of antimicrobial stewardship are to optimize antimicrobial use to improve patient outcomes and minimize adverse consequences. A successful antimicrobial stewardship program is one that is multidisciplinary. Pharmacists are core members of antimicrobial stewardship and undertake multiple roles to accomplish the goals of the program. As antimicrobial stewardship continues to expand across the patient care continuum, pharmacists will serve a vital role in preserving the armamentarium of antimicrobials and improving quality of patient care.

Optimal antimicrobial therapy must take into account the key factors in antibiotic selection, that is, spectrum, tissue penetration, resistance potential, safety profile, and relative cost-effectiveness. The least expensive drug is usually accompanied by other concerns, such as high resistance potential, poor side-effect profile, pharmacokinetic properties that limit penetration into target tissue (site of infection), and/or suboptimal activity against the presumed/known pathogen. It is false economy to preferentially select the least expensive antibiotics solely because of its acquisition cost. Therapeutic failure and hidden costs may make an apparently less expensive antibiotic most costly in the end.

Traditionally, initial antibiotic therapy was administered intravenously (IV). Over the past 3 decades, there has been increased understanding, appreciation, and application of pharmacokinetic (PK) and pharmacodynamic (PD) principles in antibiotic therapy. The utilization of PK/PD parameters as applied to antimicrobial therapy has led to optimizing dosage regimens as well as increased awareness and experience with oral versus antibiotic therapy. When an oral antibiotic, given at the same dose as its IV formulation, results in the same serum/tissue levels, then oral antibiotics should be used whenever possible. When chosen carefully, oral therapy provides many benefits over IV therapy.

Because of the increasing plague of antimicrobial resistance and antibiotic misuse, antimicrobial stewardship programs (ASPs) are now a mandatory entity in all US hospitals. ASPs can use technological advances, such as the electronic medical record and clinical decision support systems, to affect a larger patient population with more efficiency. In addition, through the use of mobile applications and social media, ASPs can highlight and propagate educational information regarding antimicrobial utilization to patients and providers in a widespread and timely manner. In this article, the authors describe how technology can play an important role in antimicrobial stewardship.

Appropriate metrics are needed to measure the quality, clinical, and financial impacts of antimicrobial stewardship programs. Metrics are typically categorized into antibiotic use measures, process measures, quality measures, costs, and clinical outcome measures. Traditionally, antimicrobial stewardship metrics have focused on antibiotic use, antibiotic costs, and process measures. With health care reform, practice should shift to focusing on clinical impact of stewardship programs over financial impact. This article reviews the various antimicrobial stewardship metrics that have been described in the literature, evidence to support these metrics, controversies surrounding metrics, and areas in which future research is necessary.

Erratum

In the July 2018 issue of *Medical Clinics* (Volume 102, Issue 4), the affiliations for Patrick G. O'Connor and Michael D. Stein are listed incorrectly. The affiliations for both editors are:

Patrick G. O'Connor, MD, MPH
    Dan Adams and Amanda Adams Professor of General Medicine
    Chief, General Internal Medicine
    Yale University School of Medicine
    Yale-New Haven Hospital
    Yale University
    New Haven, Connecticut

Michael D. Stein, MD
    Professor and Chair
    Department of Health Law, Policy, and Management
    Boston University School of Public Health
    Boston, Massachusetts

The online version of this issue has been corrected.

Med Clin N Am 102 (2018) xvii
https://doi.org/10.1016/j.mcna.2018.07.001
0025-7125/18/© 2018 Published by Elsevier Inc.

medical.theclinics.com

Foreword

Make Antibiotics Great Again

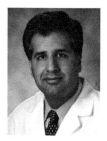

Bimal H. Ashar, MD, MBA, FACP
Consulting Editor

In 1909, German physician, Paul Ehrlich, discovered a chemical called arsphenamine that was found to be an effective treatment for syphilis.[1] This became the first modern antibiotic, with penicillin being discovered about two decades later. Today, there are well over 100 different antibiotics on the market that are being prescribed for a multitude of different symptoms/infections. According to the Centers for Disease Control and Prevention, there were approximately 269 million outpatient antibiotic prescriptions filled in 2015. An estimated 30% of these prescriptions are thought to be unnecessary.[2]

But why do physicians prescribe antibiotics so freely? There are likely numerous reasons. First, patient pressure and expectations certainly influence prescriptions. Providers want patients to be satisfied, and prescribing an antibiotic may foster that and enhance the doctor-patient relationship. Second, time constraints limit providers' ability and desire to engage in explanaions about the individual and societal risks of inappropriate antibiotic use. The path of least resistance is the easiest route to be able to get to the end of the day. Third, there is an assumption by both patients and physicians that there is little downside to prescribing and taking antibiotics and that the benefit (even if just a placebo) outweighs the risk. Yet, it is this last point that needs to be challenged. Excess antibiotic prescriptions put patients at needless risk for adverse drug reactions, including *Clostridium difficile* infections. Furthermore, the development of antibiotic resistance has made previously powerful antimicrobials virtually worthless.

It is this last point that is the subject of this issue of *Medical Clinics of North America*. Dr Cunha has enlisted infectious disease and antibiotic resistance experts from around the country to help providers become more effective stewards of antimicrobial use. If we do not, we are harming our patients as well as patients of physicians of the next generation. There are a few new antibiotic classes in the drug pipeline. If we are able to learn, incorporate, and teach judicious use of

Med Clin N Am 102 (2018) xix–xx
https://doi.org/10.1016/j.mcna.2018.06.002
0025-7125/18/© 2018 Published by Elsevier Inc.

antimicrobials, we can prolong and enhance these drugs' life-saving potential and *make antibiotics great again*!

Bimal H. Ashar, MD, MBA, FACP
Division of General Internal Medicine
Johns Hopkins University School of Medicine
601 North Caroline Street
#7143
Baltimore, MD 21287, USA

E-mail address:
Bashar1@jhmi.edu

REFERENCES

1. Tan SY, Grimes S. Paul Ehrlich (1854-1915): man with the magic bullet. Singapore Med J 2010;51(11):842–3.
2. Fleming-Dutra KE, Hersh AL, Shapiro DJ, et al. Prevalence of inappropriate antibiotic prescriptions among U.S. ambulatory care visits, 2010–2011. JAMA 2016;315:1864–73.

Preface

An Overview of Antimicrobial Stewardship Programs: Imperatives, Interventions, and Innovations

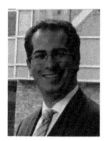

Cheston B. Cunha, MD, FACP
Editor

Antibiotic Stewardship or Antimicrobial Stewardship Programs (ASPs) are The Joint Commission (TJC) mandated to optimize antibiotic use in the hospital. Before ASPs were formally created, infectious disease (ID) clinicians were the stewards of antibiotic therapy. ID clinicians continue to be the leaders and advocates of optimal antibiotic use. Effective ASPs require a multidisciplinary coordinated approach led by a dynamic ID clinician team leader supported by a staff of ID-trained clinical PharmDs and IT personnel. Also vital is close cooperation of the microbiology laboratory and infection control and hospital epidemiology.

The ID clinician team leader should possess the requisite interpersonal, diplomatic, and leadership skills key to directing a successful ASP tailored to the institution's particular ASP problems. ASPs have their own imperatives in defining objectives and developing effective interventions. ASP interventions should be customized and prioritized to the hospital's needs. Successful early ASP efforts demonstrate effectiveness and gives confidence to administration and medical staff, which paves the way for further future ASP measures. The effectiveness of ASP interventions is best assessed by prospective audits, which guide the ASP leadership team to refine or redirect specific interventions as well as support new innovative approaches to specific ASP problem areas.

While ASP are mandated, to be maximally effective, ASPs require substantial and ongoing financial commitment from the hospital's administration. ASP is a wise hospital investment since various ASP measures will save the hospital money

Med Clin N Am 102 (2018) xxi–xxiii
https://doi.org/10.1016/j.mcna.2018.06.001
0025-7125/18/© 2018 Published by Elsevier Inc.

(eg, decreased drug costs, fewer adverse drug effects, decreased *Clostridium difficile*, decreased MDROs [Multi-drug Resistant Organisms]). Further savings come from optimal antibiotic dosing and shorter duration of therapy. The greatest cost-savings come from robust IV-to-PO switch programs, which decrease phlebitis, reduce central line–associated infections, decrease length of stay, and provide earlier discharge. The savings from IV-to-PO switch programs offset the costs of ASPs. The next step after successful IV-to-PO efforts is entirely PO antibiotic therapy, which has even more clinical and economic advantages than IV-to-PO switch programs.

Ultimately, ASP acceptance and success depend on medical staff support. The ID clinician ASP Director and Clinical ID-trained PharmD support team are critical in providing medical education on optimal antibiotic use to practitioners. Key ASP concepts can be reinforced by case consultations. Common ASP problem areas are determining appropriate spectrum by infection site, differentiating colonization (no treatment) from infection, avoiding polypharmacy when well-selected monotherapy is adequate, avoiding treating "fever and leukocytosis" as well as noninfectious febrile disorders or viral infections. The manifest advantages of IV-to-PO switch programs are impressive from an ASP perspective.

While IV-to-PO switch programs are often regarded as the "low hanging fruit" of ASPs, there are two areas that are most difficult to control (ie, antibiotic resistance problems [MDROs], *C difficile*). Controlling MDROs and *C difficile* is difficult because the factors responsible for their presence are not completely understood, making interventions particularly problematic. In some hospitals, Klebsiella pneumoniae carbapenemase (KPC) resistance seems to be related to the volume of carbapenem use, while in other hospitals, high rates of carbapenem use has had no effect on KPC rates. To further complicate the analysis, the MDRO potential varies among the carbapenems (ie, all carbapenems are not alike with respect to resistance potential). Not to mention, many MDROs isolated in hospital originate from the community (eg, chronic care facilities). Similarly, all the determinants of *C difficile* toxin production are unknown, and not simply related to antibiotic tonnage. Furthermore, antibiotics differ in their *C difficile* potential and which antibiotic is chosen matters quite a bit. Some antibiotics are protective against *C difficile* (eg, doxycycline, tigecycline). Importantly, there are a variety of non–antibiotic medications that may cause *C difficile* diarrhea (eg, proton pump inhibitors). Also needed to be considered is patient- or fomite-to-person spread.

In summary, prudent antibiotic use is the main ASP imperative. Implied in the ASP imperative are the following: monotherapy is preferred, use the shortest duration of therapy to effect cure, use optimal dose/dosing intervals to optimize PK/PD properties, do not treat fevers due to nonbacterial infections, use PO entirely whenever possible or at least IV-to-PO switch most of the time. ASP success requires enthusiastic medical staff support and antibiotic education. ASP consultations on a case-by-case basis reinforce ASP principles daily. Confidence is gained by the staff over time in experiencing firsthand the effectiveness of ASP interventions. The most challenging ASP problems (eg, MDROs and *C difficile*) will require novel innovations.

This issue of *Medical Clinics of North America* is intended for medical practitioners. The success of any ASP depends on the understanding, and enthusiastic support of the medical staff is essential. The articles in this issue were written by experts in their fields. Readers will benefit from their experience in the various aspects of ASPs. It is hoped that practitioners will find these articles of interest and practical use.

Cheston B. Cunha, MD, FACP
Antibiotic Stewardship Program
Division of Infectious Disease
Rhode Island Hospital
593 Eddy Street
Physicians Office Building
Suite #328
Providence, RI 02903, USA

E-mail address:
ccunha@lifespan.org

Antimicrobial Stewardship Programs: Principles and Practice

Cheston B. Cunha, MD

KEYWORDS

- Antimicrobial stewardship • Antibiotic therapy • Resistance • Antibiotic optimization
- C difficile

KEY POINTS

- A successful antimicrobial stewardship program (ASP) requires enthusiastic support from the administration as well as the medical staff.
- Although the core elements of successful ASPs are similar between programs, differences between hospital programs are expected and necessary given that each hospital has unique ASPs.
- The ASP must work closely with the medical staff, microbiology laboratory, and infection control to ensure optimal impact.

INTRODUCTION

Antimicrobial stewardship involves optimizing antibiotic use while using cost-effective interventions to minimize antibiotic resistance and control *Clostridium difficile*. For decades before the widespread introduction of antimicrobial stewardship programs (ASPs), infectious disease (ID) clinicians have been the antibiotic stewards in hospitals. Recently, the Centers for Disease Control and Prevention (CDC) has mandated and codified ASPs for all US hospitals.

PRINCIPLES OF ANTIMICROBIAL STEWARDSHIP PROGRAMS

The CDC has based its ASP recommendations on 7 key elements. Firstly, the hospital must designate a single ID clinician who will direct the hospital's ASP efforts. To be effective, the ID clinician leader must possess the requisite interpersonal, diplomatic, and leadership skills that are the basis for the enthusiastic support of the medical staff. The ID clinician leader should have special expertise in various aspects of antimicrobial therapy, that is, pharmacokinetics, resistance, pharmacoeconomics, and *C difficile*.[1–5]

Antibiotic Stewardship Program, Division of Infectious Disease, Rhode Island Hospital, 593 Eddy Street, Physicians Office Building, Suite #328, Providence, RI 02903, USA
E-mail address: ccunha@lifespan.org

Med Clin N Am 102 (2018) 797–803
https://doi.org/10.1016/j.mcna.2018.04.003
0025-7125/18/© 2018 Elsevier Inc. All rights reserved.

To head an effective hospital-wide ASP, the ID ASP team leader needs full and ongoing financial support for the ASP from the hospital administration. Support includes a staff of ID-trained clinical pharmacists (PharmDs), a vital component of ASPs. The ID team leader and PharmDs need committed information technology (IT) support, that is, prospective audits, data collection to track and monitor antibiotic resistance and *C difficile*, as well as ASP cost savings to the institution.[2,6]

Aside from the basics of ASPs cited earlier, a successful ASP depends on medical staff's understanding and support. Ongoing antibiotic education tailored to each clinical service's needs is essential for the acceptance of ASP interventions. The medical staff needs to understand the principles of antibiotic therapy put forth in ASP initiatives to accept and support ASP recommendations for the benefit of patients and the hospital.[1,7]

Most physicians need relevant antibiotic education to understand what constitutes optimal antimicrobial therapy, that is, pharmacokinetic/pharmacodynamic-based dosing, intravenous (IV) versus oral administration, dosing adjustments in renal/hepatic insufficiency, factors in tissue penetration, shortest duration of therapy for cure, antibiotic resistance potential, antibiotic *C difficile* potential (**Box 1**).

ASPs' success also depends on a coordinated multidisciplinary approach, which includes the critical support of the microbiology laboratory and infection control and hospital epidemiology. Antibiotic therapy has potential untoward consequences, for example, antibiotic resistance and *C difficile*; but it is equally important to recognize that control of multidrug-resistant organisms and *C difficile* are not entirely related to antibiotic factors[1,8,9] (**Box 2**).

ANTIBIOTIC MYTHS

Besides the core elements of ASPs, program effectiveness is based on other important determinants of antimicrobial therapy. In ASPs, the devil indeed is in the details.

Box 1
Effective antibiotic stewardship program

ASP leadership team
- ID clinician ASP team leader
- Clinical ID-trained PharmDs
- Tracks and reports antibiotic use
- Conduct prospective audits to assess effectiveness of ASP interventions

Antibiotic education
- Medical staff education on optimal antibiotic therapy
- Medical staff education on antibiotic resistance
- Medical staff education on antibiotic-related *C difficile*

Administration support
- ASP personnel funding
- Dedicated IT personnel funding

Liaison relationships
- Medical microbiology laboratory on resistance
- Infection control and hospital epidemiology on containment of resistance and control of *C difficile*

Box 2
Antimicrobial stewardship principles and practice: beyond the guidelines

Monotherapy versus combination therapy

- Preferably use monotherapy whenever possible to cover the most likely pathogen or cultured pathogen clinically relevant to the site of infection.

- Combination therapy should be avoided if possible. Always try to preferentially use monotherapy.

- Monotherapy is usually less expensive than combination therapy and has less potential for adverse effects and drug-drug interactions.

- Combination therapy is often used for potential synergy (rarely occurs and if used must be based on microbiology laboratory synergy studies), to increase spectrum (preferable to use monotherapy with same spectrum), or to prevent resistance (except for TB, ineffective in nearly all contributors).

Narrow- versus broad-spectrum therapy

- Narrow versus broad spectrum does not prevent resistance; for example, in treating *Escherichia coli* urosepsis, switching from a carbapenem (broad spectrum) to ampicillin (narrow spectrum) may actually increase resistance potential.

- Narrow spectrum versus broad spectrum is not clinically superior to well-chosen broad spectrum therapy; for example, switching from ceftriaxone (broad spectrum) to penicillin (narrow spectrum) in treating *Streptococcus pneumoniae* has no clinical rationale or clinical advantage and has no effect on controlling resistance.

- Antibiotic resistance is not related to spectrum narrowness or broadness, for example, levofloxacin (broad spectrum but low resistance potential) versus ampicillin (narrow spectrum but high resistance potential).

Colonization versus infection

- Treat infection, not colonization.

- Provide empirical coverage primarily directed against the most probable pathogens causing the infection at the body site.

- Avoid covering or chasing multiple organisms cultured that are not (pathogens and nonpathogens) cultured at the body site.

- Colonization of respiratory secretions, wounds, or urine with water (*Stenotrophomonas maltophilia, Burkholderia cepacia, Pseudomonas aeruginosa*) or skin organisms (MSSA, MRSA, coagulase negative Staphylococcus [CoNS], VSE, VRE) is the rule.

Antibiotic resistance

- The best way to control resistance is a selectively restricted formulary, restricted only to high-resistance-potential antibiotics, for example, imipenem (not meropenem or ertapenem), ceftazidime (not other third of fourth generation cephalosporin), and gentamicin/tobramycin (not amikacin).

- Some antibiotics may be restricted for other reasons; for example, excessive vancomycin (IV not oral) use predisposes to VRE emergence, and vancomycin may cause cell wall thickening in *Staphylococcus aureus* resulting in permeability-related resistance (to vancomycin and other antibiotics, eg, daptomycin).

- Over restriction of antibiotics may impair timely effective therapy and does not, per se, decrease resistance.

- Preferentially select antibiotics (all other things being equal) with a low resistance potential. Avoid, if possible, high-resistance-potential antibiotics, for example, macrolides (for respiratory infections) and TMP-SMX (for UTIs).

- Because resistance is, in part, concentration dependent, subtherapeutic or low antibiotic tissue concentrations (all other things being equal) predispose to resistance.

- Suboptimal dosing or usual dosing with inadequate tissue penetration, for example, into the body fluids or undrained abscesses (source control is key), predisposes to resistance.

C difficile diarrhea/colitis

- Preferentially select antibiotics (all other things being equal) with low *C difficile* potential.
- Predisposing factors to *C difficile* include relatively few antibiotics, for example, clindamycin, β-lactams, and ciprofloxacin.
- Most antibiotics have little/no *C difficile* potential, for example, aminoglycosides, aztreonam, macrolides, TMP-SMX, colistin, polymyxin B, daptomycin, Q/D, doxycycline, minocycline, tigecycline, vancomycin, and linezolid.
- Some antibiotics are protective against *C difficile*, for example, doxycycline and tigecycline.
- Always consider nonantibiotic factors that may predispose to *C difficile*, for example, cancer chemotherapy, antidepressants, statins, and PPIs.
- Also consider person-to-person spread or acquisition from the environment.

Oral and IV-to-oral switch antibiotic

- Wherever possible, treat with entirely oral antibiotic therapy instead of IV therapy.
- Switch from IV-to-oral antibiotic therapy after clinical defervescence (usually <72 hours).
- Early IV-to-oral switch therapy eliminates phlebitis and IV line–associated infections.

Pharmacoeconomic considerations

- The least expensive therapy is usually not the best therapy.
- The least expensive antibiotic (acquisition cost) may, in fact, be expensive (ie, total cost) when considering the cost implications to the institution of dosing frequency, *C difficile* potential, resistance potential, degree of activity against the known or likely pathogen, and the cost of potential therapeutic failure vis-à-vis increased LOS and medicolegally.
- Stewardship savings are best achieved by decreasing the duration of antibiotic therapy and by treating entirely with oral antibiotic therapy or early IV-to-oral switch therapy.

Abbreviations: LOS, length of stay; MRSA, methicillin-resistant *Staphylococcus aureus*; MSSA, methicillin-sensitive *Staphylococcus aureus*; PPIs, proton pump inhibitors; Q/D, quinupristin/dalfopristin; TB, tuberculosis; TMP-SMX, trimethoprim-sulfamethoxazole; UTIs, urinary tract infections; VRE, vancomycin-resistant *Enterococcus*; VSE, vancomycin-sensitive *Enterococcus*.

Adapted from Cunha CB, Cunha BA. Overview of antimicrobial therapy. In: Cunha CB, Cunha BA, editors. Antibiotic essentials. 15th edition. New Delhi (India): Jaypee Brothers Medical Publishers; 2017. p. 13–6; with permission.

Antibiotic myths and misconceptions abound. All too often, antibiotic therapy is regarded as a cure-all for all febrile disorders. As long as patients are covered with one or more antibiotics, all will be well. Multiple antibiotics (polypharmacy) are the rule when carefully selected monotherapy is optimal. Polypharmacy is nearly always unnecessary and increases costs and increases the potential of adverse events. Excluding a very few examples, combination therapy does not provide synergy or prevent resistance.

COLONIZATION VERSUS INFECTION

A daily problem for practitioners is to differentiate colonization from actual infection. Colonization, of course, should not be treated. Most physicians feel compelled to treat any organism cultured from body sites. Only infection need be treated. Needlessly treating colonization wastes resources and sets the stage for resistance and/or *C difficile* problems.

ANTIBIOTIC RESISTANCE DETERMINANTS

Contrary to popular belief, most resistance in hospital comes from the community, for example, nursing homes, chronic care facilities, and the food supply (antibiotics are commonly used in foods). In the hospital, every effort should be made to not worsen resistance by preferential selection of low-resistance-potential antibiotics. There are many misconceptions about resistance, that is, resistance is class related, related to volume, or related to duration of use. Practically, antibiotics may be considered as having a low or high resistance potential. The low-resistance-potential antibiotics, for example, doxycycline, induce little or no resistance independent of volume or duration of use. In contrast, high-resistance-potential antibiotics, for example, ampicillin, may induce resistance even with limited use and are likely to cause even more resistance if used in high volume. Within each antibiotic class are low- and high-resistance-potential antibiotics, for example, among third-generation cephalosporins, ceftazidime has a high resistance potential, whereas ceftriaxone has a low resistance potential, an example that resistance is not related, per se, to antibiotic class[2,8,10] (**Table 1**).

CLOSTRIDIUM DIFFICILE DIARRHEA

Another difficult ASP challenge is *C difficile* diarrhea (CDD). It is widely thought that *C difficile* is antibiotic related. Also, it is not appreciated that antibiotic *C difficile* potential, like antibiotic resistance potential, differs among antibiotics. Clindamycin and beta lactams (excluding ceftriaxone) are the most frequent antibiotic causes of CDD. Most other antibiotics have low *C difficile* potential, for example, macrolides, tetracyclines, aztreonam, aminoglycosides, and trimethoprim-sulfamethoxazole. Some antibiotics are actually protective against *C difficile*, for example, doxycycline, tigecycline. In selecting an antibiotic, practitioners should consider *C difficile* potential as well as resistance potential.

CLINICAL AND PHARMACOECONOMIC BENEFITS

Optimal antibiotic therapy is based on the aforementioned principles, but other ASP interventions benefit the patients and the hospital, that is, IV-to-oral switch therapy. The advantages of IV-to-oral switch are important in decreasing drug costs (oral antibiotics cost less, at any given dose, than their IV equivalents) as well as decreasing the incidence of phlebitis (shorter duration of IV lines). As importantly, IV-to-oral switch programs increase patient satisfaction (shorter IV days and earlier discharge) and decrease the hospital length of stay.[1,11,12]

Importantly, although ASPs are now mandated, sustained funding from the administration and enthusiastic medical staff support are needed for program success. The cost savings to the hospital from IV-to-oral switch programs offset the costs of ASPs.

PRACTICE OF ANTIMICROBIAL STEWARDSHIP PROGRAMS

ASPs necessarily must differ among hospitals because hospitals differ in size, location (rural, suburban, urban), teaching (vs community), staff antibiotic prescribing habits, presence or absence of full-time ID clinicians, resistance patterns, and so forth. Clearly, one size does not fit all.

What is a successful ASP intervention in one hospital is ineffective in another. The ASP ID team leader and clinical ID-trained PharmD staff are responsible for customizing ASP interventions to the hospital's unique set of antibiotic use–related concerns. The effectiveness of various ASP interventions are assessed and modified based on

Table 1
Resistance potential of selected antibiotics

High-Resistance-Potential Antibiotics to Avoid	Usual Organisms Resistance to Each Antibiotic	Preferred Low-Resistance-Potential Antibiotic Alternatives in Same Class	Preferred Low-Resistance-Potential Antibiotic Alternatives in Different Classes
Aminoglycosides			
Gentamicin or tobramycin	Pseudomonas aeruginosa	Amikacin	Levofloxacin, colistin, cefepime
Cephalosporins			
Ceftazidime	Pseudomonas aeruginosa	Cefepime	Levofloxacin, colistin, polymyxin B
Tetracyclines			
Tetracycline	Streptococcus pneumoniae	Doxycycline, minocycline	Levofloxacin, moxifloxacin
Quinolones			
Ciprofloxacin	Streptococcus pneumoniae	Levofloxacin, moxifloxacin	Doxycycline
Ciprofloxacin	Pseudomonas aeruginosa	Levofloxacin	Amikacin, colistin, cefepime
Glycopeptides			
Vancomycin	MSSA MRSA	None	Linezolid, daptomycin, minocycline, tigecycline
Carbapenems			
Imipenem	Pseudomonas aeruginosa	Meropenem, doripenem	Amikacin, cefepime, colistin, polymyxin B
Macrolides			
Azithromycin	Streptococcus pneumoniae	None	Doxycycline, levofloxacin, moxifloxacin
Dihydrofolate			
Reductase inhibitors			
TMP-SMX	Streptococcus pneumoniae	None	Doxycycline, levofloxacin, moxifloxacin

Abbreviations: MRSA, methicillin-resistant *Staphylococcus aureus*; MSSA, methicillin-sensitive *Staphylococcus aureus*; TMP-SMX, trimethoprim-sulfamethoxazole.

the findings from prospective audits. Prospective audits identify ineffective interventions and may suggest modifications or entirely new innovative approaches.[1,13–17]

REFERENCES

1. Cunha CB. Principles of antimicrobial stewardship. In: LaPlante KL, Cunha CB, Morrill HJ, et al, editors. Antimicrobial stewardship: principles and practice. London: CABI Press; 2017. p. 1–8.
2. Cunha BA, Hage JE, Schoch PE, et al. Overview of antimicrobial therapy. In: Cunha CB, Cunha BA, editors. Antibiotic essentials. 15th edition. New Delhi (India): Jaypee Brothers Medical Publishers Ltd; 2017. p. 1–16.
3. Carling P, Fung T, Killion A, et al. Favorable impact of a multidisciplinary antibiotic management program conducted during 7 years. Infect Control Hosp Epidemiol 2003;24:699–706.

4. Doron S, Davidson LE. Antimicrobial stewardship. Mayo Clin Proc 2011;86: 1113–23.

5. Wagner B, Filice GA, Drekonja D, et al. Antimicrobial stewardship programs in inpatient hospital settings: a systematic review. Infect Control Hosp Epidemiol 2014;35:1209–28.

6. MacDougall C, Polk RE. Antimicrobial stewardship programs in health care systems. Clin Microbiol Rev 2005;18:638–56.

7. Salsgiver E, Bernstein D, Simon MS, et al. Knowledge, attitudes and practices regarding antimicrobial use and stewardship among prescribers at acute-care hospitals. Infect Control Hosp Epidemiol 2018;39:316–22.

8. Schechner V, Temkin E, Harbarth S, et al. Epidemiological interpretation of studies examining the effect of antibiotic usage on resistance. Clin Microbiol Rev 2013;26:289–307.

9. Fraser GL, Stogsdill P, Dickens JD Jr, et al. Antibiotic optimization. An evaluation of patient safety and economic outcomes. Arch Intern Med 1997;157:1689–94.

10. Cunha BA. Effective antibiotic-resistance control strategies. Lancet 2001;357: 1307–8.

11. Cyriac JM, James E. Switch over from intravenous to oral therapy: a concise overview. J Pharmacol Pharmacother 2014;5:83–7.

12. McCallum AD, Sutherland RK, Mackintosh CL. Improving antimicrobial prescribing: implementation of an antimicrobial i.v.-to-oral switch policy. J R Coll Physicians Edinb 2013;43:294–300.

13. Nowak MA, Nelson RE, Breidenbach JL, et al. Clinical and economic outcomes of a prospective antimicrobial stewardship program. Am J Health Syst Pharm 2012; 69:1500–8.

14. John JF Jr, Fishman NO. Programmatic role of the infectious diseases physician in controlling antimicrobial costs in the hospital. Clin Infect Dis 1997;24:471–85.

15. Ruttimann S, Keck B, Hartmeier C, et al. Long-term antibiotic cost savings from a comprehensive intervention program in a medical department of a university-affiliated teaching hospital. Clin Infect Dis 2004;38:348–56.

16. Ohl CA, Luther VP. Health care provider education as a tool to enhance antibiotic stewardship practices. Infect Dis Clin North Am 2014;28:177–93.

17. Cunha CB, Varughese CA, Mylonakis E. Antimicrobial stewardship programs (ASPs): the devil is in the details. Virulence 2013;4:147–9.

Antimicrobial Stewardship and Antimicrobial Resistance

Louis B. Rice, MD

KEYWORDS

- Antimicrobial resistance • Antimicrobial stewardship • Interventions
- Antimicrobial restriction • Antimicrobial cycling • Decision support

KEY POINTS

- Antimicrobial stewardship programs over the years have had several goals, including reducing costs, optimizing therapeutic outcomes, and reducing antimicrobial resistance. Reductions of antimicrobial resistance have been the most elusive.
- The relationship between antimicrobial usage and resistance is also not always direct, especially with molecular mechanisms that confer resistance to multiple classes of antibiotics or through transferable plasmids and transposons that contain multiple resistance genes.
- The understanding of which techniques are most effective is limited by the fact that many studies are descriptive or quasiexperimental.
- More recently, several meta-analyses or systematic reviews of stewardship programs have been published, offering encouragement that some interventions, especially those that involve prospective auditing and feedback, have the effect of reducing overall antimicrobial selective pressure, and are associated with infection control interventions, can have an important impact on resistance rates in individual institutions.

INTRODUCTION

Since the concept of antimicrobial stewardship was introduced by McGowan and Finland[1] and others in the 1970s, stewardship programs have evolved from cost-containment exercises to efforts to optimize the treatment of infections (primarily in hospitals) and more recently to decrease the antimicrobial selective pressure that promotes the emergence and spread of antimicrobial resistance. Stewardship programs' track records of decreasing antimicrobial costs have been generally positive, using in many cases preapproval programs that promote the use of less expensive antimicrobial alternatives.[2] Strategies designed to optimize the treatment of infections have

Department of Medicine, Warren Alpert Medical School of Brown University, Rhode Island Hospital, 593 Eddy Street, Providence, RI 02903, USA
E-mail address: lrice@lifespan.org

Med Clin N Am 102 (2018) 805–818
https://doi.org/10.1016/j.mcna.2018.04.004
0025-7125/18/© 2018 Elsevier Inc. All rights reserved.

generally used computer programs that offer advice on appropriate dosing of infections relative to the patient,[3] such as programs that recommend appropriate adjustments of antimicrobial doses in patients with renal failure, in pediatric patients, or in patients with larger than normal body masses. Such programs may also recommend optimal dosing based on commonly accepted pharmacodynamic principles, such as the killing parameters for a given antibiotic class (concentration-dependent killing, time-dependent killing, or area under the curve calculations). Examples of the beneficial effects of these types of pharmacodynamic analyses include the use of aminoglycosides in a single daily dose (optimizing killing and minimizing toxicity)[4] or the development of daptomycin as a single daily dose antibiotic.[5] Other recommendations based on pharmacodynamic data, such as the use of β–lactam agents as a continuous infusion, have not been widely demonstrated to result in improved outcomes in the clinical setting, but may be useful for critically ill patient with sepsis with respiratory infections.[6]

Comprehensive programs designed to minimize overall antimicrobial resistance are recent and take their cues in some cases from previous examples of outbreaks of resistant bacteria that have been successfully controlled by limiting the use of a particular class of agents. We discuss several examples of such strategies later in this article, but it is first important to delineate some general definitions and principles relevant to the relationship between antimicrobial use and resistance. **Table 1** lists six principles that should be kept in mind when evaluating any stewardship strategies.

HISTORICAL BASES FOR BELIEF THAT STEWARDSHIP CAN CONTROL ANTIMICROBIAL RESISTANCE

Although it is sometimes said that there would not be antimicrobial resistance without the use of antibiotics, this sentiment is not strictly true. It is known, for example, that gram-negative bacilli are intrinsically resistant to vancomycin, presumably because the large vancomycin molecule cannot traverse the porins of the gram-negative outer membrane. Similarly, anaerobic bacteria are resistant to aminoglycosides because the movement of aminoglycosides across the cytoplasmic membrane is an oxygen-dependent process. We do not formally consider these resistance phenotypes to be problems because they are considered the natural spectrum of the antibiotic in question. Resistance is considered a problem when it occurs in bacteria normally within an antibiotic's spectrum of activity, such as *Escherichia coli* resistance to ampicillin, *Pseudomonas aeruginosa* resistance to imipenem, *Staphylococcus aureus* resistance to oxacillin, or *Enterococcus faecium* resistance to vancomycin. In such instances, increasing levels of resistance are virtually always associated with use of one or more classes of antibiotics.

The association between use and resistance is sometimes interpreted as causation, and with good reason. Most antibiotics have broad spectra of activity. Use of these antibiotics invariably alters the flora of the person who is taking them, creating a circumstance where resistant bacteria have a selective advantage for growth. The emergence and spread of resistant bacteria logically occurs in settings where this selective advantage is present. It is also sometimes claimed that resistant bacteria are at a selective disadvantage because expressing resistance has some metabolic cost, either because of the energy required to replicate a resistance plasmid or activate an efflux pump, or because of the compromised function of a target protein that has mutated to resistance, or metabolic disadvantages that result from the loss of normal functions of porins or efflux pumps. In some cases, selective disadvantages are demonstrated in growth experiments comparing mutated with wild-type strains.

Table 1
Important concepts when thinking about antimicrobial resistance in nosocomial pathogens

Concept	Explanation
Some resistance mechanisms (β-lactamases, topoisomerase mutations, membrane charge alterations) are specific to a given antibiotic or class of antibiotics, whereas others (reductions of porins, activation of multidrug efflux pumps) represent either general defense or detoxification mechanisms.	This distinction is important, because the first type of mechanism may be counteracted by using an antibiotic with a different mechanism of action, but the second is more likely to make the strain resistant to a variety of unrelated agents. The mechanism may therefore be selected by a variety of antibiotics and confer resistance to antibiotics other than the class that selected.
In most cases, resistant mutants are selected, not created.	Mutations occur constantly in replicating bacteria. Among bacteria that have the capacity to exchange genes, either with members of their own species or even other species, gene exchange is also regularly occurring. Administering antibiotics creates an environment where strains that express resistance have a selective advantage over those that do not. Antibiotics inhibit the growth of bacteria that lack resistance, hence facilitating the emergence of those that do express it.
Resistance commonly emerges distant from the site of infection.	With a few exceptions, such as the emergence of cephalosporin resistance during *Enterobacter cloacae* bacteremia[46] or the emergence of *Pseudomonas aeruginosa* resistance to virtually any antibiotic in a high-inoculum infection,[32] the emergence of resistance on therapy among common nosocomial or community-acquired pathogens at the site of infection is rare. More commonly, resistance emerges among strains colonizing other parts of the body, such as the gastrointestinal tract, respiratory tract, the perineal area, or areas of the skin. Such resistance is often selected from the flora present in the environment, which in many hospitals is replete with resistant strains of many species.
Pharmacodynamic principles are helpful in recommending appropriate dosing strategies to maximize treatment success but are rarely relevant in preventing the emergence of resistance.	One concept that has emerged from pharmacodynamics principles is that of the mutant prevention concentration, which is that concentration of antibiotic that exceeds the minimal inhibitory concentration required to prevent growth of the most resistant first-order mutant to a given antibiotic. Even in the laboratory, this strategy only works for antibiotics for whom resistance occurs in a gradual and graded fashion, such as the fluoroquinolones. The strategy is moot for resistance phenotypes in which single point mutations of relevant genes result in minimal inhibitory concentration orders of magnitude greater than the susceptible strain (as with rifampin resistance) or for acquired genes (eg, β-lactamases), which can also dramatically increase resistance. Moreover, resistance frequently occurs at sites distant from the site of infection, where antimicrobial concentrations vary considerably. Fluoroquinolones have been shown to rapidly select resistant strains on the skin, in the pharynx, and in the gastrointestinal tract.

(continued on next page)

Table 1
(continued)

Concept	Explanation
Combinations of antibiotics do not prevent the emergence of resistance in nosocomial pathogens.	The concept of using combinations of antibiotics to prevent the emergence of resistance to either agent alone is derived from early experience treating tuberculosis, where patients responded miraculously to streptomycin therapy, only to return a few months later with recurrent disease, now resistant to streptomycin. Combination therapy has been highly successful at eradicating infection and preventing resistance in tuberculosis. Similar principles have proven effective in treating human immunodeficiency virus. The commonality between these two pathogens is that their only route to resistance is target alteration through genomic mutation. Routine nosocomial pathogens, in contrast, often exchange large amounts of DNA with other strains in, among other places, the gastrointestinal tract. They can acquire multiple resistance genes to a variety of antibiotics in a single exchange. Under these circumstances, adding more antibiotic INCREASES the likelihood that a multiresistant strain emerges.
The concepts of "narrowing down" therapeutic regimens are flawed.	Antibiotics are commonly referred to as either narrow in their spectrum (eg, ampicillin) or broad in their spectrum (eg, imipenem). This distinction is made because imipenem has clinically important activity against more of the pathogens that are confronted in the hospital (eg, *Klebsiella pneumoniae, E cloacae,* or *P aeruginosa*). Yet in the hospital setting, activity against competing flora may be of prime importance in the selection of multiresistant strains. Ampicillin is broadly active against virtually all streptococcal species, which are prominent components of the gastrointestinal tract. It is also active against a wide variety of anaerobes and many gram-negative aerobic and facultative species. It is susceptible to hydrolysis by most β-lactamases, including the KPC-type enzymes that hydrolyze carbapenems. It is far from certain that ampicillin would not select KPC-producing bacteria in a clinical environment where these enzymes are prevalent. The only truly convincing narrowing of anti-gram-negative therapy is stopping antibiotics entirely.

However, growth disadvantages cannot always be demonstrated in resistant strains, and animal experiments designed to investigate the fate of impaired resistance phenotypes show that compensatory mutations restoring growth abilities to the resistant bacteria often occur in nonselective environments, rather than mutation back to susceptibility.[7]

Despite these concerns, it makes sense that reducing selective pressure associated with antibiotic use will ameliorate a resistance problem in a circumscribed system, such as a hospital, and even in the community. Several studies have provided support for this presumption. Among the earliest studies was an interesting report from a neurologic intensive care unit in Scotland, published in 1966.[8] Because of a problem of postoperative wound infections caused by S aureus and antibiotic-sensitive coliforms, prophylactic therapy with ampicillin and cloxacillin was used for selected patients in the unit. The following year several colonizations and infections with resistant Klebsiella aerogenes were noted, including one fatal case of meningitis. The problem persisted despite movement to an entirely new geographic unit. Movement of infected patients to a separate unit and treatment with very high doses of colistin led to some therapeutic successes, but did not abort the outbreak, which was accompanied by widespread environmental contamination. The supervisors of the unit finally took the drastic measure of discontinuing the use of all prophylactic and therapeutic antibiotics. The investigators were gratified to observe not only a dramatic reduction in the prevalence of infection and colonization by resistant Klebsiella, but a 60% to 70% reduction in the rate of all infections in the unit.

The 1980s were characterized by the clinical introduction of a variety of third-generation cephalosporins. These agents (principally cefotaxime, ceftizoxime, ceftriaxone, and ceftazidime) had activity against pathogens, such as Enterobacter spp, Citrobacter freundii, and, in the case of ceftazidime, P aeruginosa, which were characteristically resistant to other available β-lactams. The widespread use of these agents was associated with the emergence and spread of gram-negative bacilli, most commonly Klebsiella pneumoniae, which were resistant by expressing extended-spectrum β-lactamases (ESBLs).[9] The first versions of these enzymes contained one or more amino acid substitutions in the common narrow-spectrum β-lactamases TEM and SHV that resulted in the ability to hydrolyze extended-spectrum cephalosporins. These amino acid substitutions commonly had the effect of "opening up" the active site of the enzyme, allowing it to accommodate the cephalosporins and their bulky side chains. Most of these mutant enzymes became more susceptible to inhibition by the clinically available β-lactamase inhibitors, but that susceptibility was soon overcome by the overexpression of several different β-lactamases by these strains.[10]

Many efforts to abort ESBL outbreaks by using strict infection control efforts had limited success, with several studies suggesting that ESBL-producing bacteria were endemic and polyclonal and therefore not demonstrably the result of transfer from one patient to the next by health care workers.[11,12] The failure of infection control measures led to efforts to control ESBL outbreaks by controlling the amount of cephalosporins used, which by and large were successful.[13,14] Of course, by the 1990s no one was willing to outlaw all antibiotics as they had in Scotland three decades earlier, so a different class of antibiotics had to be substituted for the cephalosporins. In most cases the antibiotic that was substituted in was either a carbapenem or piperacillin-tazobactam. Both substitution strategies met with gratifying success in reducing ESBL-producing K pneumoniae, suggesting that it was the reduction in the selective pressure of cephalosporins that was the important component of the intervention strategy, and not the nature of the substituted antibiotic. In some cases, overuse of the carbapenems was associated with subsequent outbreaks of carbapenem-resistant species, leading the late Jim Rahal to suggest the compelling "squeezing the balloon" analogy to characterize attempts to use antibiotic switches to control resistance.[15]

Most of the efforts to control resistance in gram-positive bacteria in the first few decades of antimicrobial usage centered on controlling methicillin-resistant S aureus (MRSA). The first MRSA outbreaks occurred in European hospitals in the 1960s and were controlled primarily by strict infection control regimens.[16] S aureus is a pathogen that colonizes skin surfaces and the upper respiratory tract in humans, and many of the early outbreaks were believed to be caused by the clonal spread of strains through the hospital, so it was logical that strict infection control measures would be critical to its control. That S aureus was also subject to the selective pressures of antimicrobial administration was brought into stark relief in the late 1980s with the clinical introduction of ciprofloxacin. When introduced, ciprofloxacin was touted as the first orally administered antimicrobial agent effective for the treatment of MRSA.[17] In vitro activities were excellent and clinical trials were supportive. Remarkably, at many hospitals throughout the United States resistance rates to ciprofloxacin for MRSA increased from less than 10% to greater than 70% in less than 2 years.[18] Ciprofloxacin and other fluoroquinolones achieve significant concentrations throughout the body, including the skin and anterior nares.[19] Clinical studies showed that nasal colonization by fluoroquinolone-resistant staphylococci was observed within days of oral antimicrobial administration.[19,20] Whether controlling fluoroquinolone usage will exert a significant impact on rates of MRSA colonization in high-prevalence settings remains an open question.

Two other significant nosocomial pathogens for whom antimicrobial associations with gastrointestinal colonization and subsequent infection have been important are vancomycin-resistant E faecium (VRE) and Clostridium difficile. Although associations of VRE outbreaks with vancomycin usage have been reported, associations have also been found with heavy use of cephalosporins and agents that have potent activity against anaerobic bacteria. Animal studies have suggested that cephalosporins that are concentrated in the gastrointestinal tract (eg, ceftriaxone) promote the establishment of VRE gastrointestinal colonization (ie, increasing the susceptibility of the person to colonization),[21] whereas agents with potent antianaerobic activity dramatically increase the number of VRE present in the stool (increasing the likelihood of further cross-transmission).[22] At least one human study has confirmed that exposure to agents with potent antianaerobic activity significantly increases the quantities of VRE detectable in stool cultures.[23] Reductions in the use of extended-spectrum cephalosporins have resulted in improvements in VRE colonization rates in some small studies.[24]

C difficile infection has been associated with the use of virtually any antibiotic, but all antibiotics are not created equal in terms of their association with C difficile. Shortly after the discovery of C difficile as the cause of antibiotic-associated diarrhea and pseudomembranous colitis, exposure to clindamycin was identified as a major risk factor.[25] Subsequent work revealed that the strain associated with several early outbreaks expressed a constitutively expressed ermB gene, conferring resistance to clindamycin.[26] Subsequent studies have identified cephalosporins as significant risk factors for C difficile infection, possibly because C difficile are intrinsically resistant to cephalosporins.[25] More recently, C difficile infection has been closely tied to the use of fluoroquinolones, presumably because the more recent predominant strains have mutations in their topoisomerase genes conferring resistant to this class of agents.[27] Studies have reported reductions in rates of C difficile associated with controlling the use of clindamycin, cephalosporins, and fluoroquinolones.[25]

Reports of associations between antibiotic use and resistance in the community have been sporadic. One important study showed a substantial reduction in the rates of erythromycin resistance in Streptococcus pyogenes in Finland associated with overall reductions of macrolide use in that country over a period of 5 to 7 years.[28] However, Bean and colleagues[28] reported no change in the incidence of sulfa resistance in E coli despite a 97% reduction in sulfa use in the United Kingdom from 1991 to 1999.

ANTIMICROBIAL STEWARDSHIP TECHNIQUES

The tools available for the antimicrobial stewardship teams in hospitals include limiting formularies and formal restrictions of certain classes of antimicrobials, the cycling of antibiotics; and decision support, including prospective audit and feedback and, as an important component of any program, education of the prescribing staff.

Antimicrobial Restriction

Limiting antimicrobial formularies and restricting the use of certain antibiotics is a technique that has been used for decades. In many cases, the limitations have been dictated by cost, with the motivation to decrease the overall hospital spend on antibiotics. In general, because newer drugs tended to be more expensive than older drugs, and having a broader spectrum of activity, these practices in effect resulted in promoting more narrow-spectrum alternatives. In a 1974 study, McGowan and Finland[1] reviewed the use of antibiotics in Boston City Hospital. Although antibiotics were generally freely available to all prescribers, an antibiotic usage committee designated certain antimicrobials as restricted, meaning that the prescriber needed to consult with (although not officially obtain the approval of) a designated infectious diseases physician before using the antibiotic. Restricted antibiotics included those "whose potential for toxicity or for causing emergence of resistance among organisms prevalent in the hospital or whose high cost warrant some restriction on their use." Even with this lax policy, use of ampicillin moved from an average of 7127 g per year during the 3 years when it was restricted 62,613 g per year for the 4 years of unrestricted use. Conversely, chloramphenicol's move from the unrestricted to the restricted list was associated with a reduction in its use from more than 20,000 g/y before restriction to an average of 2900 g/y while it was restricted.

McGowan and Finland[1] did not include data on susceptibility patterns associated with their changes in antibiotic usage. Recco and colleagues[2] attempt to replicate McGowan and Finland's work at Coney Island Hospital showed a roughly 50% reduction in their use of antibiotics, especially their use of cephalosporins. This reduction was associated with an increase in the rates of cephalothin-resistant E coli, however, likely attributed to the fact that the reduction in cephalothin use was accompanied by an increase in the use of intravenous ampicillin, which would be expected to select for some of the same resistance mechanisms.

Clearly, placing even small hurdles for doctors prescribing antibiotics can have a major impact on their practices and changed prescribing practices can have significant, if at times unpredictable, effects on antibiotic susceptibility patterns. In the setting of an outbreak of ESBL-producing K pneumoniae, restriction of cephalosporins can have a significant impact on the prevalence of that type of resistance in an institution, if use is replaced by an antibiotic without similar selection tendencies. Moreover, in the absence of a specific outbreak it is not clear which antimicrobial agents should be restricted to minimize resistance. Any policy that merely replaces overuse of one class of antibiotics for another is likely to run into further resistance problems down the road.[29]

Antimicrobial Cycling

Antimicrobial cycling, or "crop rotation," refers to practices in which there are predetermined changes in empirical usage of antibiotics, usually within a certain unit of a hospital, that occur according to a prespecified time schedule. The goal is to avoid prolonged use of a single class of antibiotics and thereby the selection of resistance to that class. In general, such programs that occur in intensive care units, for example, might rotate an extended-spectrum cephalosporin, such as cefepime, with a carbapenem, piperacillin-tazobactam, and depending on local susceptibilities, a fluoroquinolone. There are practical problems with such a strategy, including inconvenience ("which antibiotic are we prescribing this month?"), determining optimal cycle length, defining the geographic reach of the cycling strategy, baseline resistance issues, and periodic antibiotic shortages. There are also theoretic reasons why cycling may not work. The first is that some resistance phenotypes may be selected by a variety of antibiotics. Vancomycin-resistant enterococci are as likely to be selected by antianaerobic agents or cephalosporins as by vancomycin[30,31]; imipenem-resistant *P aeruginosa* can be selected by ciprofloxacin,[32] and ESBL-producing *K pneumoniae* are likely to be resistant to β-lactam/β-lactamase inhibitor combinations.[10] A second theoretic problem is that many of the resistance mechanisms selected by different classes of antibiotics are not specific, but rather general detoxification mechanisms (pump activations, porin reductions) and therefore are as likely to confer resistance against the antibiotic of the next cycle and the current antibiotic.

Still, it is worth looking at the data to determine whether cycling holds promise on a larger scale. Early results were not encouraging, prompting Marin Kollef of Washington University of St. Louis and a prominent clinical researcher in the area, to state: "Unfortunately, the cumulative evidence to date suggests that antibiotic cycling has limited efficacy for preventing antibiotic resistance."[33] However, more recently some meta-analyses have suggestive more reason for optimism. Baur and colleagues[34] performed a meta-analysis of studies examining the effect of antibiotic stewardship on the incidence of infection and colonization with multiresistant bacteria and *C difficile* and concluded, based on three studies, that antimicrobial cycling was the "most effective" of the stewardship interventions. It is worth looking in more detail at the three studies on which this conclusion was based.

The bulk of the conclusion was based on a study by Chong and colleagues,[35] which used a cycling strategy in a closed hematologic malignancy unit. The cycling involved rotating, monthly, the antibiotic used for empiric treatment of febrile neutropenia among cefepime, piperacillin-tazobactam, meropenem, and ciprofloxacin. In the pre-rotation period, cefepime was the standard therapy used for febrile neutropenia, and the investigators were concerned about a rising incidence of ESBL-producing, cefepime-resistant *E coli*. The intervention, which was followed for 20 months, was associated with a statistically significant reduction in the rate of cefepime-resistant, ESBL-producing gram-negative isolates in the blood and a statistically significant reduction in the rate of cefepime-resistant *E coli* fecal colonization. Overall cefepime use in the unit, which was 45% of the total of the four antibiotics in rotation before the rotation started, was reduced to 9.3% of the total and there was a 63% reduction in total quantity of cefepime administered. Piperacillin-tazobactam administration, which represented 32% of the total before the rotation period, increased to 76% of the total in the final rotation period. Given these data, it is fair to ask whether the operative intervention was a replacement of cefepime by piperacillin-tazobactam or the rotation of the different antibiotics.

A second study cited by Baur and colleagues[34] was published by Smith and colleagues,[36] who looked at the impact of a strategy in which linezolid was alternated every 3 months with vancomycin for the empirical treatment of suspected gram-positive infections in a single intensive care unit. During the cycling period, the investigators saw a statistically significant reduction in the percentage of staphylococcal infections that were caused by MRSA, although there was no reduction in the overall incidence of S aureus infections in the unit. There was also no change in the rate off VRE infections (the primary end point of the study as originally designed). Because it is hard to find a logical explanation for the effect on the MRSA infection rate but not the methicillin-sensitive S aureus infection rate by rotating these two drugs, the ultimate implications of this study are not clear.

In a study published by Takesue and colleagues,[37] a whole-hospital program was instituted in which antimicrobial use was constantly monitored and evaluated, and every 3 months antibiotics were categorized as restricted (during which use was discouraged by the stewardship team), recommended (during which use was encouraged by the stewardship team), or off supervision (no recommendation either way). Antibiotics were placed into the different categories based on the previous 3 months of usage data and antimicrobial susceptibility results. The intervention was associated with a gradual decline in the isolates of resistant gram-negative bacilli and of resistant P aeruginosa. Overall, a significantly greater degree of antimicrobial heterogeneity was observed in the intervention period.

It is difficult to draw firm conclusions regarding the cost-benefit of antimicrobial cycling strategies from these three studies. The Chong study seems to be yet another example of a cephalosporin for piperacillin-tazobactam switch resulting in reduction in the occurrence of infections caused by ESBL-producers. The Takesue study is impressive in their effort to look at antimicrobial usage and susceptibility rates in real time and adjust based on that, but that is not really a formal cycling program. The Smith study has a firm conclusion regarding MRSA incidence, but confusing and perhaps conflicting results with methicillin-sensitive S aureus and VRE. Given the logistical difficulties of implementing formal cycling protocols across large areas of the hospital, it would seem a worthwhile effort to find other means of achieving antimicrobial heterogeneity.

Abel zur Wiesch and colleagues[38] performed a separate meta-analysis of cycling studies, including 11 studies (among them the Chong and Smith studies described previously). They concluded based on their analysis that cycling programs are effective in reducing overall infections and resistant infections. They then developed a theoretic model of adjustable cycling/mixing in which they assume that antimicrobial therapies will be changed if initial therapy is ineffective. Cycling (which was predicted to be detrimental if a strict regimen was used) under this model was predicted to be beneficial in suppressing single and especially multiple resistance. The period they used for cycling was 1 month, speculating that longer periods may be detrimental.

Decision Support, Including Prospective Audit and Feedback

Efforts to provide physicians with the knowledge and tools to appropriately prescribe antimicrobial agents in the hospital have existed since the advent of the electronic medical record. In 1996, Pestotnik and colleagues[3] published their experience with designing and implementing an antibiotic management program within their electronic medical record at Latter Day Saints Hospital in Salt Lake City, Utah. The critical aspect of this program was that the designers made a point to engage the relevant stakeholders before rolling out the program. This buy-in was critical to the success of the program. The program provided guidance on prophylactic, empirical, and therapeutic use of antibiotics in the context of individual and institutional antimicrobial resistance patterns and offered advice on appropriate antimicrobial dosing considering modifying factors, such as renal function and prior adverse reactions. Analysis of the effect of the program showed marked improvements in the use of prophylactic antibiotics, significant reductions in the number of adverse reactions associated with antibiotic administration, and stable rates of susceptibility in important gram-negative pathogens.

A more recent report from Spain[39] described encouraging results of an educational antimicrobial stewardship program on hospital-acquired candidemia and multidrug-resistant isolates. This program involved peer-to-peer educational interviews between counselors and providers. A set of clinical guidelines developed by 64 representatives from different clinical departments and coordinated by the infectious diseases team was used as the basis for the educational interventions. The educational interventions were conducted according to a schedule determined by each department's level of antibiotic consumption and were patient-based. The most frequent interventions were for inappropriate lengths of therapy (52.8%) and for inappropriate choice of agent (38.6%). Within the first year of the program, inappropriate use of antibiotics declined, as did the overall usage of antibiotics within the institution. Usage of cephalosporins and fluoroquinolones declined by approximately one-third. This trend persisted over the 5-years of the study,[40] during which the investigators also noted a highly significant reduction in the incidence of infections caused by hospital-acquired *Candida* spp and by multidrug-resistant gram-negatives, along with a concomitant reduction in the mortality rate attributable to multidrug-resistant organisms.

META-ANALYSES OF STEWARDSHIP PROGRAMS AND ANTIBIOTIC RESISTANCE

Several meta-analyses and systematic reviews of antimicrobial stewardship programs have recently been published. Although their conclusions differed in detail, all found that stewardship programs were effective in reducing the nosocomial occurrence of infections caused by resistant bacteria. Feazel and colleagues[41] included 16 publications and found a 52% reduction in the incidence of *C difficile* infections after introduction of an antimicrobial stewardship program. Karanika and colleagues,[42] in contrast, did not find a relative risk reduction for *C difficile* infections associated with stewardship in seven articles, none of which were included in the Feazel review. They did find relative risk reductions for infections caused by MRSA, imipenem-resistant *P aeruginosa*, and ESBL-producing *K pneumoniae*. Davey and colleagues[43] reviewed 221 studies and concluded with high certainty that stewardship interventions increase compliance with antibiotics policies and reduce duration of antibiotic treatment by more than 1 day. They do not seem to increase mortality and may reduce the overall length of hospital stay. They may reduce infections caused by *C difficile*, but evidence for that was believed to be weak. Finally, Schuts and colleagues[44] reviewed 145 studies and found that six process interventions (empirical therapy according to guidelines, de-escalation of therapy, intravenous to oral switch, therapeutic drug monitoring, use of a list of restricted antibiotics, and bedside consultation) showed some benefit on one or more of four predetermined outcomes (clinical outcomes, adverse effects, cost, and bacterial resistance rates). Resistance rates were reduced in association with restrictions on antibiotics.

Baur and colleagues[34] reviewed 32 studies looking specifically for impact on the incidence of infection and colonization with antibiotic-resistant bacteria and *C difficile*. They found significant reductions for multiresistant gram-negative bacteria, ESBL-producing gram-negative bacteria, MRSA, and *C difficile*, but no difference with incidence of vancomycin-resistant enterococci, and fluoroquinolone- and aminoglycoside-resistant gram-negative bacteria. Importantly, they found that stewardship interventions are more effective when implemented along with infection control measures.

SUMMARY

The understanding of the effectiveness of stewardship interventions has been inhibited by the weaknesses of study designs to date (generally before/after or quasiexperimental) and the variety of interventions that have been used. Still the preponderance of the evidence suggests that such programs are safe and can have beneficial effects on costs, toxicities, and antimicrobial resistance rates. The salutary effects arise from two different stewardship results: reductions in overall antimicrobial usage and increased heterogeneity of antibiotics used. Of these two results, the more important is to reduce overall antimicrobial usage, thereby decreasing the selective pressure for resistance. Increasing heterogeneity without reducing overall consumption may work in specific settings, such as outbreaks of ESBL-producing *K pneumoniae* where cephalosporins are reduced in favor of piperacillin-tazobactam or a carbapenem, but this success often proves a pyrrhic victory because other resistance phenotypes eventually emerge. The recent dramatic success reported by Molina and colleagues[40] resulting from their educational stewardship intervention suggests that the best way forward is to engage prescribing physicians and educate them in a patient-specific way about the proper use of antibiotics, ideally with as much hard evidence on risks and benefits as can be mustered. Whether surrogate markers of infection, such as procalcitonin, which in a recent meta-analysis[45] was shown to reduce mortality and antibiotic exposure in the treatment of acute respiratory infections, should become a standard component of stewardship programs remains an open question that should be studied.

REFERENCES

1. McGowan JE Jr, Finland M. Usage of antibiotics in a general hospital: effect of requiring justification. J Infect Dis 1974;130(2):165–8.
2. Recco RA, Gladstone JL, Friedman SA, et al. Antibiotic control in a municipal hospital. JAMA 1979;241(21):2283–6.
3. Pestotnik SL, Classen DC, Evans RS, et al. Implementing antibiotic practice guidelines through computer-assisted decision support: clinical and financial outcomes. Ann Intern Med 1996;124(10):884–90.
4. Nicolau DP, Wu AH, Finocchiaro S, et al. Once-daily aminoglycoside dosing: impact on requests and costs for therapeutic drug monitoring. Ther Drug Monit 1996;18(3):263–6.
5. Oleson FB Jr, Berman CL, Kirkpatrick JB, et al. Once-daily dosing in dogs optimizes daptomycin safety. Antimicrob Agents Chemother 2000;44(11):2948–53.
6. Vardakas KZ, Voulgaris GL, Maliaros A, et al. Prolonged versus short-term intravenous infusion of antipseudomonal beta-lactams for patients with sepsis: a systematic review and meta-analysis of randomised trials. Lancet Infect Dis 2018; 18(1):108–20.

7. Bjorkman J, Nagaev I, Berg OG, et al. Effects of environment on compensatory mutations to ameliorate costs of antibiotic resistance. Science 2000;287(5457): 1479–82.

8. Price DJ, Sleigh JD. Control of infection due to *Klebsiella aerogenes* in a neurosurgical unit by withdrawal of all antibiotics. Lancet 1970;2(7685):1213–5.

9. Bush K. Classification of ß-lactamases: groups 1, 2a, 2b and 2b'. Antimicrob Agents Chemother 1989;33:264–70.

10. Essack SY, Hall LM, Pillay DG, et al. Complexity and diversity of *Klebsiella pneumoniae* strains with extended-spectrum beta-lactamases isolated in 1994 and 1996 at a teaching hospital in Durban, South Africa. Antimicrob Agents Chemother 2001;45(1):88–95.

11. Harris AD, Kotetishvili M, Shurland S, et al. How important is patient-to-patient transmission in extended-spectrum beta-lactamase *Escherichia coli* acquisition. Am J Infect Control 2007;35(2):97–101.

12. Johnson JK, Smith G, Lee MS, et al. The role of patient-to-patient transmission in the acquisition of imipenem-resistant *Pseudomonas aeruginosa* colonization in the intensive care unit. J Infect Dis 2009;200(6):900–5.

13. Meyer KS, Urban C, Eagan JA, et al. Nosocomial outbreak of *Klebsiella* infection resistant to late-generation cephalosporins. Ann Intern Med 1993;119:353–8.

14. Rice LB, Eckstein EC, DeVente J, et al. Ceftazidime-resistant *Klebsiella pneumoniae* isolates recovered at the Cleveland Department of Veterans Affairs Medical Center. Clin Infect Dis 1996;23:118–24.

15. Rahal JJ, Urban C, Segal-Maurer S. Nosocomial antibiotic resistance in multiple gram-negative species: experience at one hospital with squeezing the resistance balloon at multiple sites. Clin Infect Dis 2002;34(4):499–503.

16. Michel MF, Priem CC. Control at hospital level of infections by methicillin-resistant staphylococci in children. J Hyg (Lond) 1971;69(3):453–60.

17. Piercy EA, Barbaro D, Luby JP, et al. Ciprofloxacin for methicillin-resistant *Staphylococcus aureus* infections. Antimicrob Agents Chemother 1989;33:128–30.

18. Raviglione MC, Boyle JF, Mariuz P, et al. Ciprofloxacin-resistant methicillin-resistant *Staphylococcus aureus* in an acute care hospital. Antimicrob Agents Chemother 1990;34:2050–4.

19. Hoiby N, Jarlov JO, Kemp M, et al. Excretion of ciprofloxacin in sweat and multiresistant *Staphylococcus epidermidis*. Lancet 1997;349(9046):167–9.

20. Peterson LR, Quick JN, Jensen B, et al. Emergence of ciprofloxacin resistance in nosocomial methicillin-resistant *Staphylococcus aureus* isolates. Resistance during ciprofloxacin plus rifampin therapy for methicillin-resistant *S aureus* colonization. Arch Intern Med 1990;150(10):2151–5.

21. Donskey CJ, Hanrahan JA, Hutton RA, et al. Effect of parenteral antibiotic administration on establishment of colonization with vancomycin-resistant *Enterococcus faecium* in the mouse gastrointestinal tract. J Infect Dis 2000;181:1830–3.

22. Donskey CJ, Hanrahan JA, Hutton RA, et al. Effect of parenteral antibiotic administration on persistence of vancomycin-resistant *Enterococcus faecium* in the mouse gastrointestinal tract. J Infect Dis 1999;180:384–90.

23. Donskey CJ, Chowdhry TK, Hecker MT, et al. Effect of antibiotic therapy on the density of vancomycin-resistant enterococci in the stool of colonized patients. N Engl J Med 2000;343(26):1925–32.

24. Quale J, Landman D, Saurina G, et al. Manipulation of a hospital antimicrobial formulary to control an outbreak of vancomycin-resistant enterococci. Clin Infect Dis 1996;23:1020–5.

25. Owens RC Jr, Donskey CJ, Gaynes RP, et al. Antimicrobial-associated risk factors for *Clostridium difficile* infection. Clin Infect Dis 2008;46(Suppl 1):S19–31.

26. Johnson S, Samore MH, Farrow KA, et al. Epidemics of diarrhea caused by a clindamycin-resistant strain of *Clostridium difficile* in four hospitals. N Engl J Med 1999;341(22):1645–51.

27. McDonald LC, Killgore GE, Thompson A, et al. An epidemic, toxin gene-variant strain of *Clostridium difficile*. N Engl J Med 2005;353(23):2433–41.

28. Bean DC, Livermore DM, Papa I, et al. Resistance among Escherichia coli to sulphonamides and other antimicrobials now little used in man. J Antimicrob Chemother 2005;56(5):962–4.

29. Rahal JJ, Urban C, Horn D, et al. Class restriction of cephalosporin use to control total cephalosporin resistance in nosocomial *Klebsiella*. J Am Med Assoc 1998; 280:1233–7.

30. Donskey CJ, Schreiber JR, Jacobs MR, et al. A polyclonal outbreak of predominantly VanB vancomycin-resistant enterococci in Northeast Ohio. Clin Infect Dis 1999;29(3):573–9.

31. Padiglione AA, Wolfe R, Grabsch EA, et al. Risk factors for new detection of vancomycin-resistant enterococci in acute-care hospitals that employ strict infection control procedures. Antimicrob Agents Chemother 2003;47(8):2492–8.

32. Aubert G, Pozzetto B, Dorche G. Emergence of quinolone-imipenem cross-resistance in *Pseudomonas aeruginosa* after fluoroquinolone therapy. J Antimicrob Chemother 1992;29(3):307–12.

33. Kollef MH. Is antibiotic cycling the answer to preventing the emergence of bacterial resistance in the intensive care unit? Clin Infect Dis 2006;43(Suppl 2):S82–8.

34. Baur D, Gladstone BP, Burkert F, et al. Effect of antibiotic stewardship on the incidence of infection and colonisation with antibiotic-resistant bacteria and *Clostridium difficile* infection: a systematic review and meta-analysis. Lancet Infect Dis 2017;17(9):990–1001.

35. Chong Y, Shimoda S, Yakushiji H, et al. Antibiotic rotation for febrile neutropenic patients with hematological malignancies: clinical significance of antibiotic heterogeneity. PLoS One 2013;8(1):e54190.

36. Smith RL, Evans HL, Chong TW, et al. Reduction in rates of methicillin-resistant *Staphylococcus aureus* infection after introduction of quarterly linezolid-vancomycin cycling in a surgical intensive care unit. Surg Infect (Larchmt) 2008;9(4):423–31.

37. Takesue Y, Nakajima K, Ichiki K, et al. Impact of a hospital-wide programme of heterogeneous antibiotic use on the development of antibiotic-resistant gram-negative bacteria. J Hosp Infect 2010;75(1):28–32.

38. Abel zur Wiesch P, Kouyos R, Abel S, et al. Cycling empirical antibiotic therapy in hospitals: meta-analysis and models. PLoS Pathog 2014;10(6):e1004225.

39. Cisneros JM, Neth O, Gil-Navarro MV, et al. Global impact of an educational antimicrobial stewardship programme on prescribing practice in a tertiary hospital centre. Clin Microbiol Infect 2014;20(1):82–8.

40. Molina J, Penalva G, Gil-Navarro MV, et al. Long-term impact of an educational antimicrobial stewardship program on hospital-acquired candidemia and multidrug-resistant bloodstream infections: a quasi-experimental study of interrupted time-series analysis. Clin Infect Dis 2017;65(12):1992–9.

41. Feazel LM, Malhotra A, Perencevich EN, et al. Effect of antibiotic stewardship programmes on *Clostridium difficile* incidence: a systematic review and meta-analysis. J Antimicrob Chemother 2014;69(7):1748–54.

42. Karanika S, Paudel S, Grigoras C, et al. Systematic review and meta-analysis of clinical and economic outcomes from the implementation of hospital-based anti-microbial stewardship programs. Antimicrob Agents Chemother 2016;60(8): 4840–52.

43. Davey P, Marwick CA, Scott CL, et al. Interventions to improve antibiotic prescribing practices for hospital inpatients. Cochrane Database Syst Rev 2017;(2):CD003543.

44. Schuts EC, Hulscher M, Mouton JW, et al. Current evidence on hospital antimicrobial stewardship objectives: a systematic review and meta-analysis. Lancet Infect Dis 2016;16(7):847–56.

45. Schuetz P, Wirz Y, Sager R, et al. Effect of procalcitonin-guided antibiotic treatment on mortality in acute respiratory infections: a patient level meta-analysis. Lancet Infect Dis 2018;18(1):95–107.

46. Chow JW, Fine MJ, Shlaes DM, et al. *Enterobacter* bacteremia: clinical features and emergence of antibiotic resistance during therapy. Ann Intern Med 1991; 115:585–90.

Antimicrobial Resistance
An Antimicrobial/Diagnostic Stewardship and Infection Prevention Approach

Edward Joel Septimus, MD

KEYWORDS

- Antimicrobial resistance • Antimicrobial stewardship • Diagnostic stewardship
- De-escalation • Audit and feedback

KEY POINTS

- Antimicrobial resistance (AR) is one of the most serious public health threats today, which has been accelerated by the overuse and misuse of antimicrobials in humans and animals plus inadequate infection prevention.
- Antimicrobial stewardship refers to a collaborative, multidisciplinary program designed to improve antimicrobial prescribing to optimize clinical outcomes while minimizing unintended consequences of antimicrobial use, such as toxicity, selection of pathogenic organisms, and emergence of resistance.
- The accurate and timely microbiology provided by the laboratory supports the application of medical knowledge and judgment to achieve the best outcomes for patients with an infectious disease, especially in an era of increased AR.
- Interventions include audit and feedback with or without preauthorization. De-escalation and prescribing an antibiotic for the appropriate duration are important components as well.
- A multipronged approach is necessary combining human and animal stewardship, preventions of health care–associated infections, development of new vaccines, and better diagnostic testing.

INTRODUCTION

Antimicrobial resistance (AR) is one of the most serious public health threats today, which has been accelerated by the overuse and misuse of antimicrobials in humans and animals plus inadequate infection prevention (IP) measures.[1] Numerous studies have shown a relationship between antimicrobial use and resistance.[2,3] The increasing incidence of multidrug-resistant organism (MDRO) infections has become a safety concern for patients across the continuum of patient care, especially in patients in the intensive care unit (ICU) who develop a health care–associated infection (HAI).

No conflicts.

Texas A&M College of Medicine, 4257 Albans Street, Houston, TX 77005, USA

E-mail address: eseptimus@gmail.com

Med Clin N Am 102 (2018) 819–829
https://doi.org/10.1016/j.mcna.2018.04.005
medical.theclinics.com

MRDO infections are more difficult to treat, incur greater treatment costs, and have greater morbidity and mortality than infections caused by organisms susceptible to antibiotics. Unlike other medications, the misuse of antibiotics can adversely impact the health of patients who have not received them. The human and economic cost of AR in the United States was revealed in the Centers for Disease Control and Prevention (CDC) report, *Antibiotic Resistance Threats in the United States, 2013.*[4] Using conservative estimates, the CDC determined that antibiotic resistant organisms are responsible for more than 2 million infections and 23,000 deaths per year in the United States in 2008, at a direct cost of $20 billion with additional loss to society for lost productivity as high as $35 billion per year. In 2014 a report commissioned by the Prime Minister of the United Kingdom and the Wellcome Trust projected that without global action, 10 million deaths from AR infections will occur worldwide by 2050.

Furthermore, antibiotic misuse and overuse not only facilitates the development of MDROs but they also increase unintended consequences, such as *Clostridium difficile* infections (CDIs) and antibiotic-associated adverse drug events (ADEs), making antimicrobial stewardship (AS) an important component of HAI prevention.[5] A recent meta-analysis showed AS programs reduced the incidence of infections and colonization with multidrug-resistant gram-negative bacteria, extended-spectrum β-lactamase–producing gram-negative bacteria, methicillin-resistant *Staphylococcus aureus*, as well as the incidence of CDI infections. The same study emphasized that AS programs, when implemented alongside infection control measures, especially hand-hygiene interventions, were more effective than implementation of AS alone confirming that a well-functioning IP program is a key component to a successful AS strategy.[6] Similar data have also shown that the addition of AS interventions can enhance results of robust IP measures, particularly when addressing an outbreak.[7]

AS refers to a collaborative, multidisciplinary program designed to improve antimicrobial prescribing (right drug, dose, duration, and route of administration when antibiotics are needed) to optimize clinical outcomes while minimizing unintended consequences of antimicrobial use, such as toxicity, selection of pathogenic organisms, and emergence of resistance.[8,9]

AS programs have been shown to improve patient outcomes, reduce antimicrobial adverse events, and decrease AR.[6,10] The CDC published core elements associated with successful AS programs: 7 elements for hospitals and long-term care facilities[11,12] and 4 elements for outpatient facilities.[13] These elements provide a framework for implementation. For acute care and long-term care, the 7 elements include leadership commitment, accountability, drug expertise, action, tracking, reporting, and education. For outpatient facilities, the 4 core elements include commitment, action of policy and practice, tracking and reporting, and education and expertise. Common to all 3 are the following:

1. Leadership commitment dedicating necessary human, financial, and information technology resources
2. Drug expertise
3. Tracking and reporting offering regular feedback to clinicians to improve prescribing behavior
4. Education providing educational resources to clinicians and patients on antibiotic prescribing

PREVENTION

There is a synergy between IP and AS in reducing AR. Targeted coordination and prevention strategies are critical to stopping the spread of MDROs. The use of prevention bundles has been shown to reduce HAI rates. Several studies have demonstrated the impact of catheter insertion and maintenance bundles on central line–associated bloodstream infection (CLABSI) rates and have shown that CLABSI prevention bundles are effective, sustainable, and cost-effective for both adults and children. Bundles have also been used in successful multifaceted efforts to reduce ventilator-associated pneumonia (VAP), catheter-associated urinary tract infections, and surgical site infections.[14] Recently, several studies have shown chlorhexidine gluconate (CHG) bathing in ICUs can reduce HAIs.[15,16] There has been a shift from a vertical approach targeting a single organism to a horizontal approach to reduce infections from all pathogens. CHG bathing aligns with this horizontal approach and has become the standard of care in the adult ICU in the United States.[5] Active surveillance has been advocated to identify patients who are asymptomatic with targeted MDROs, which can serve as a reservoir for transmission. For example, active surveillance has been shown to decrease colonization pressure and limit the spread of carbapenem-resistant *Enterobacteriaceae* (CRE).[17] In addition, because CRE colonization is a risk factor for CRE infection, active surveillance may identify patients at risk for CRE infections and reduce the delay in ordering appropriate antimicrobial therapy. In the end, reducing infections will result in decreased antimicrobial use resulting in decreased adverse events and lower AR.

DIAGNOSTIC STEWARDSHIP

The diagnosis of infection in critically ill patients is important because early appropriate antimicrobial therapy improves outcomes.[18] The accurate and timely microbiology provided by the laboratory supports the application of medical knowledge and judgment to achieve the best outcomes for patients with an infectious disease, especially in an era of increased AR. The laboratory provides information to help determine if patients are infected, what the pathogen is, and in most cases the susceptibility of the organism.[19] The impact of proper specimen collection is key in providing clinicians accurate information to improve patient outcomes. The clinician needs to have confidence that the results are accurate, clinically relevant, and significant.[20] Cultures should be collected before starting antibiotics whenever possible and labeled properly. Specimens of poor quality should be rejected. Specimens from body sites close to mucosal surfaces or open wounds where organisms can contaminate cultures, such as superficial wounds/ulcers/drains, fistulas, sputum, and nasal sinuses, should be carefully collected or avoided. Swab specimens should be discouraged. Actual aspirates, fluids, or tissue are preferred. The accuracy of swabs for wound cultures is only around 50% compared with biopsy or tissue collection.[21] Unjustified ordering or improper collection of urine for urinalysis and/or culture can result in overdiagnosis and overtreatment, increasing risk of antimicrobial resistance, side effects, and CDI.[22] Urine testing should only be done when urinary symptoms present, such as fever, urgency, dysuria, suprapubic and/or costovertebral tenderness, and altered mental status without another cause. Guidelines published by the Infectious Diseases Society of America (IDSA) recommend urine testing in the absence of urinary symptoms for only 2 groups: pregnant women and patients undergoing an invasive urinary procedure, such as a urologic procedure for which mucosal bleeding is likely to occur or transurethral resection of the prostate.[23] Recent studies have demonstrated that urine results, not symptoms, are driving unnecessary antibiotic use, which will accelerate resistance.[24]

Blood cultures are also a critical tool to diagnose bacteremia and guide antimicrobial therapy, especially with the increasing threat of MDROs. The volume of blood drawn for each febrile illness is important in improving detection of bacteria and candida with bloodstream infections. For adults, 20 to 30 mL of blood per culture set is recommended usually in 2 bottles, one aerobic and one anaerobic. For children, volume is based on age and weight. Additionally, in adults, 2 to 4 blood culture sets is adequate in evaluating each febrile episode.[25] Because blood is considered a sterile body fluid, anything that grows may be considered significant. However, contamination of blood cultures is still a common problem and may represent up to 25% of all positive blood cultures.[26] Contamination can lead to unnecessary antimicrobial therapy, unnecessary removal of central lines, unnecessary testing, increased length of stay, and increased cost. This leads to an increased risk of complications, such as allergic reactions, increased antimicrobial resistance, and an increased risk of CDI.[22] Interventions that have been studied to reduce contamination include disinfection methods for skin preparation with either chlorhexidine or iodine tincture, disinfecting the septum of the blood culture bottle with alcohol, and the use of dedicated phlebotomy teams.[27]

Procalcitonin (PCT) is a biomarker that has emerged as a useful laboratory test in stewardship. PCT is a calcitonin-related gene product expressed by human epithelial cells in response to bacterial infections and is conversely downregulated during viral infections.[28] In addition, studies have shown that PCT concentrations tend to decrease rapidly during improvement from acute bacterial infections.[29]

PCT has been assessed for its role in shortening the duration of antibiotic therapy for bacterial infection based on serial measurements of PCT levels and avoidance of the initiation of antibiotic therapy when the PCT level is low. Trials assessing PCT-guided discontinuation of antibiotic therapy report significantly more antibiotic-free days (2–4 days) in the PCT arm, without a negative effect on mortality.[30,31] In a recent single-center trial, the addition of PCT resulted in a significant reduction in antibiotic use and improvement in hospital mortality, 30-day readmission, CDI during hospitalization, and antimicrobial ADEs during hospitalization.[32] In a recent meta-analysis, Schuetz and colleagues[33] used PCT to guide antibiotic treatment in patients with acute respiratory infections. They showed PCT reduces antibiotic exposure and side effects and improves survival. Finally, Chu and colleagues[34] conducted a retrospective cohort on practice patterns and outcomes associated with the use of PCT in critically ill patients with sepsis. They found PCT use among critically ill patients with sepsis in real-world settings was not associated with decreased antibiotic use or improved antibiotic-associated outcomes. Importantly, PCT was measured inconsistently and often only checked once, suggesting that PCT was not implemented according to evidenced-based protocols found efficacious in other clinical trials.

Recent advances in molecular diagnostic technologies have significantly reduced the delay in infectious disease diagnosis, can identify and precisely characterize emerging pathogens and resistance genes, and trace the source of outbreaks in a manner of days.[35] To be effective, molecular diagnostic technologies must be integrated into AS.

ANTIMICROBIAL STEWARDSHIP

It is generally accepted that an appropriate antimicrobial should be started as soon as an infection is identified in critically ill patients.[18] One of the greatest challenges imposed by infections due to suspected MDROs is how to prescribe broad-spectrum therapy to cover the most likely pathogens and balance efficacy and collateral damage. AS has been proposed to enable better choices and to reduce unintended consequences, including AR.

AS programs have been shown to improve patient outcomes, reduce antimicrobial adverse events, and decrease AR.[10,36] In 2016, the IDSA and the Society for Healthcare Epidemiologists of America (SHEA) published an updated guidelines on implementing an AS program.[8] The guidelines recommends both prospective audit and feedback (AF) and preauthorization because these interventions been shown to improve antibiotic use and are recommended as core components of any stewardship program. AF interventions have also been shown to improve antibiotic use, reduce antibiotic resistance, and reduce CDI rates[37,38] without a negative impact on patient outcomes. For example, in an interrupted time-series trial, targeted ICU patients on broad-spectrum antibiotics were reviewed with AF on day 3 and day 10 of therapy. This study was conducted over a 1-year period. They reported a reduction in broad-spectrum use resulting in a 23% reduction in costs, improved gram-negative susceptibility to meropenem, and reduced CDI ($P = .04$). There was no impact on mortality compared with controls.[39]

Preauthorization is a strategy to improve antibiotic use by requiring clinicians to get approval for certain antibiotics before they are administered. Outcome studies with preauthorization have shown decreased antibiotic use and decreased antibiotic resistance, particularly among gram-negative pathogens as well as significant reduction in costs of the restricted drug.[40,41]

However, many studies use a combination of AF and preauthorization with or without IP strategies. Baur and colleagues[6] published a systemic review and meta-analysis on the effect of stewardship on the incidence of infection and colonization with resistant bacteria and CDI. They included 32 studies. which confirmed that AS programs reduced the incidence of infections and colonization with multidrug-resistant gram-negative bacteria (51% reduction; incidence rate 0.49, 95% confidence interval [CI] 0.35–0.68; $P<.0001$), extended-spectrum β-lactamase–producing gram-negative bacteria (48%; 0.52, 0.27–0.98; $P = .0428$), and methicillin-resistant *Staphylococcus aureus* (37%; 0.63, 0.45–0.88; $P = .0065$), as well as the incidence of CDI (32%; 0.68, 0.53–0.88; $P = .0029$).

Even if an appropriate initial antibiotic is selected, patient outcomes may not be assured if drug concentrations are not delivered to the site of the infection. Dosed optimization can be characterized as administering the correct antimicrobial agent and dose aimed at attaining the pharmacokinetics/pharmacodynamics (PK/PD) target for the drug given. The Surviving Sepsis Campaign's (SSC) guidelines recommend adopting dosing strategies based on accepted PK/PD principles.[42] This recommendation is important for both concentration-dependent drugs as well as time-dependent bacterial killing.[43] With time-dependent antibiotics, such as β-lactams, the optimal response occurs when the drug concentration stays greater than the mean inhibitory concentration of the organism. In contrast, in concentration-dependent antibiotics, such as aminoglycosides, the best response occurs based on peak concentration. This approach has been recommended especially in critically ill patients. Dosing strategies based on PK/PD principles for aminoglycosides, such as once-daily dosing, have been shown to be effective in reducing nephrotoxicity and improved clinical outcomes.[44] For β-lactam antibiotics, one meta-analysis showed decreased mortality (risk ratio, 0.59; 95% CI 0.41–0.83) among patients receiving continuous infusions of carbapenems or piperacillin-tazobactam versus standard infusions.[45] However, another meta-analysis did not support improved outcomes using prolonged infusions of broad-spectrum β-lactam antibiotics.[46] The SSC's guideline recommends optimizing vancomycin PK/PD in septic patients by achieving targeted trough levels by using a loading dose.[42] The impact of dose optimization and antimicrobial resistance is unclear.

De-escalation is another key strategy. De-escalation can be defined as modification of the initial empirical antimicrobial regimen based on culture results, other laboratory tests, and the clinical status of patients. The goals of de-escalation are shown in **Box 1**. Studies have demonstrated that de-escalation is performed in less than half

---

Box 1
Goals of de-escalation

- Changing from a broad-spectrum antibiotic to one with a narrower spectrum if appropriate
- Eliminating overlapping or unnecessary combination therapy targeting causative organism
- Stopping antimicrobial therapy when a noninfectious cause most likely
- Administering antimicrobial therapy for the correct duration
- Decreasing antimicrobial exposure → reduce adverse events
- Cost savings

---

of patients in whom it was deemed to be appropriate.[47] In addition, several studies have shown the mortality rate was significantly lower among patients in whom therapy was appropriately de-escalated.[48,49]

Two approaches have been suggested an antibiotic time out[50] and a day 3 bundle.[51] Both approaches suggest physicians take time to review the dose, duration, and indication when cultures and new information are available 48 to 72 hours after initiation of empirical therapy. **Box 2** reviews a checklist for an antibiotic time out. **Box 3** outlines key process measures for the day 3 bundle.

Along with reviewing empirical antibiotics at 48 to 72 hours, IDSA and SHEA also recommend that AS implement guidelines and strategies to reduce antibiotic therapy to the shortest effective duration.[8] Evidence from systematic reviews[52] and randomized controlled trials (RCTs)[53,54] have demonstrated that stewardship interventions aimed at shorter courses of antibiotic therapy for select clinical syndromes is associated with outcomes similar to those with longer courses in both adults and children with fewer adverse events. Studies support that reduction in exposure of antibiotics can decrease drug resistance, decrease cost, improve adherence, and decrease adverse events.[54] The following are a few examples. Historically, VAP has been treated for 14 to 21 days. In a multicenter RCT, Chastre and colleagues[53] demonstrated that patients who received antibiotics for 8 days had similar outcomes compared with patients who received it for 15 days for VAP. Current guidelines from the Surgical Infection Society and the IDSA recommend use of antibiotics in the treatment of complicated intra-abdominal infections for only 4 to 7 days with adequate source control instead of the traditional 10 to 14 days.[55] Lastly, RCTs have shown that treatment for 5 days can be as effective as longer treatment courses for the treatment of patients with community-acquired pneumonia (CAP). Dunbar and colleagues[56] demonstrated in a multicenter, randomized, double-blind trial that levofloxacin 750 mg per day for 5 days was at least as effective as 500 mg of levofloxacin per day for 10 days for treatment of mild to severe CAP.

Box 2
Checklist of an antibiotic time out

- Do patients have an infection that will respond to antibiotics?
- If so, are patients on the right antibiotic, dose, and route?
- Can a more targeted antibiotic be used to treat the infection (de-escalation)?
- How long should patients receive the antibiotic?

Box 3
Key process measures for the day 3 bundle

- Was there an antibiotic plan (name, dose, route, interval of administration, and planned duration)?
- Was there a review of the diagnosis?
- If positive microbiological results were available, was there any adaption of the antibiotic treatment, for example, de-escalation?
- If patients were initially started on intravenous (IV) antibiotic therapy, was the possibility of IV-oral switch documented?

From Pulcini C, Defres S, Aggarwal I, et al. Design of a 'day 3 bundle' to improve the reassessment of inpatient empirical antibiotic prescriptions. J Antimicrob Chemother 2008;61(6):1385; with permission.

Another important intervention often overlooked is improving AS in animals. Up to 80% of all antibiotics sold in the United States are administered to food animals, primarily for growth promotion and infection prophylaxis.[57] Studies have shown high rates of antibiotic resistance in the intestinal flora of farm animals and farmers and recent molecular methods have confirmed that resistant bacteria in animals are consumed by humans resulting in infection.[58] Furthermore, antibiotics used in animals are excreted in urine and stools and can disperse in fertilizer, groundwater, and surface runoff with significant impact on the environmental microbiome.[58]

Lastly, beyond the traditional AS approaches, behavioral change strategies to influence prescriber practices have been underutilized. Future AS efforts should use behavioral theory to improve intervention and sustainability.[59]

SUMMARY

In summary, antibiotic resistance is a global challenge. To address the challenge, both human and veterinary medicine must apply practical interventions, evaluate and improve stewardship programs, identify and institute best practices, and develop key communication messages for practitioners, patients, and the public. A multipronged approach is necessary combining human and animal stewardship, preventions of HAIs, development of new vaccines, and better diagnostic testing.

REFERENCES

1. Huttner A, Harbarth S, Carlet J, et al. Antimicrobial resistance: a global view from the 2013 World Healthcare-Associated Infections Forum. Antimicrob Resist Infect Control 2013;2:31.
2. Bell BG, Schellevis F, Stobberingh E, et al. A systematic review and meta-analysis of the effects of antibiotic consumption on antibiotic resistance. BMC Infect Dis 2014;14:13.
3. Goossens H. Antibiotic consumption and link to resistance. Clin Microbiol Infect 2009;15(Suppl 3):12–5.
4. Centers for Disease Control and Prevention. Antibiotic resistance threats in the United States 2013. Available at: http://www.cdc.gov/drugresistance/pdf/ar-threats-2013-508.pdf. Accessed September 12, 2017.
5. Septimus E, Weinstein RA, Perl TM, et al. Approaches for preventing healthcare-associated infections: go long or go wide? Infect Control Hosp Epidemiol 2014; 35(7):797–801.

6. Baur D, Gladstone BP, Burkert F, et al. Effect of antibiotic stewardship on the incidence of infection and colonisation with antibiotic-resistant bacteria and Clostridium difficile infection: a systematic review and meta-analysis. Lancet Infect Dis 2017;17(9):990–1001.

7. Valiquette L, Cossette B, Garant MP, et al. Impact of a reduction in the use of high-risk antibiotics on the course of an epidemic of Clostridium difficile-associated disease caused by the hypervirulent NAP1/027 strain. Clin Infect Dis 2007;45(Suppl 2):S112–21.

8. Barlam TF, Cosgrove SE, Abbo LM, et al. Implementing an antibiotic stewardship program: guidelines by the Infectious Diseases Society of America and the Society for Healthcare Epidemiology of America. Clin Infect Dis 2016;62(10):e51–77.

9. Dellit TH, Owens RC, McGowan JE Jr, et al. Infectious Diseases Society of America and the Society for Healthcare Epidemiology of America guidelines for developing an institutional program to enhance antimicrobial stewardship. Clin Infect Dis 2007;44(2):159–77.

10. Kelly AA, Jones MM, Echevarria KL, et al. A report of the efforts of the Veterans Health Administration national antimicrobial stewardship initiative. Infect Control Hosp Epidemiol 2017;38(5):513–20.

11. Centers for Disease Control and Prevention. Core elements of hospital antibiotic stewardship programs. Available at: https://www.cdc.gov/antibiotic-use/healthcare/pdfs/core-elements.pdf. Accessed August 11, 2017.

12. Centers for Disease Control and Prevention. Core elements of antibiotic stewardship programs for nursing homes. Available at: https://www.cdc.gov/longtermcare/prevention/antibiotic-stewardship.html. Accessed August 11, 2017.

13. Centers for Disease Control and Prevention. Core elements of outpatient antibiotic stewardship. Available at: https://www.cdc.gov/getsmart/community/pdfs/16_268900-a_coreelementsoutpatient_508.pdf. Accessed August 11, 2017.

14. Septimus E, Yokoe DS, Weinstein RA, et al. Maintaining the momentum of change: the role of the 2014 updates to the compendium in preventing healthcare-associated infections. Infect Control Hosp Epidemiol 2014;35(5):460–3.

15. Climo MW, Yokoe DS, Warren DK, et al. Effect of daily chlorhexidine bathing on hospital-acquired infection. N Engl J Med 2013;368(6):533–42.

16. Huang SS, Septimus E, Platt R. Targeted decolonization to prevent ICU infections. N Engl J Med 2013;369(15):1470–1.

17. Schwaber MJ, Carmeli Y. An ongoing national intervention to contain the spread of carbapenem-resistant enterobacteriaceae. Clin Infect Dis 2014;58(5):697–703.

18. Ferrer R, Martin-Loeches I, Phillips G, et al. Empiric antibiotic treatment reduces mortality in severe sepsis and septic shock from the first hour: results from a guideline-based performance improvement program. Crit Care Med 2014;42(8):1749–55.

19. Dik JW, Poelman R, Friedrich AW, et al. An integrated stewardship model: antimicrobial, infection prevention and diagnostic (AID). Future Microbiol 2016;11(1):93–102.

20. Morency-Potvin P, Schwartz DN, Weinstein RA. Antimicrobial stewardship: how the microbiology laboratory can right the ship. Clin Microbiol Rev 2017;30(1):381–407.

21. Stevens DL, Bisno AL, Chambers HF, et al. Practice guidelines for the diagnosis and management of skin and soft-tissue infections. Clin Infect Dis 2005;41(10):1373–406.

22. Fridkin S, Baggs J, Fagan R, et al. Vital signs: improving antibiotic use among hospitalized patients. MMWR Morb Mortal Wkly Rep 2014;63(9):194–200.

23. Hooton TM, Bradley SF, Cardenas DD, et al. Diagnosis, prevention, and treatment of catheter-associated urinary tract infection in adults: 2009 International Clinical Practice Guidelines from the Infectious Diseases Society of America. Clin Infect Dis 2010;50(5):625–63.

24. Pallin DJ, Ronan C, Montazeri K, et al. Urinalysis in acute care of adults: pitfalls in testing and interpreting results. Open Forum Infect Dis 2014;1(1):ofu019.

25. Cockerill FR 3rd, Wilson JW, Vetter EA, et al. Optimal testing parameters for blood cultures. Clin Infect Dis 2004;38(12):1724–30.

26. Weinstein MP. Blood culture contamination: persisting problems and partial progress. J Clin Microbiol 2003;41(6):2275–8.

27. Hall KK, Lyman JA. Updated review of blood culture contamination. Clin Microbiol Rev 2006;19(4):788–802.

28. Schuetz P, Albrich W, Mueller B. Procalcitonin for diagnosis of infection and guide to antibiotic decisions: past, present and future. BMC Med 2011;9:107.

29. Charles PE, Tinel C, Barbar S, et al. Procalcitonin kinetics within the first days of sepsis: relationship with the appropriateness of antibiotic therapy and the outcome. Crit Care 2009;13(2):R38.

30. Bouadma L, Luyt CE, Tubach F, et al. Use of procalcitonin to reduce patients' exposure to antibiotics in intensive care units (PRORATA trial): a multicentre randomised controlled trial. Lancet 2010;375(9713):463–74.

31. Nobre V, Harbarth S, Graf JD, et al. Use of procalcitonin to shorten antibiotic treatment duration in septic patients: a randomized trial. Am J Respir Crit Care Med 2008;177(5):498–505.

32. Broyles MR. Impact of procalcitonin-guided antibiotic management on antibiotic exposure and outcomes: real-world evidence. Open Forum Infect Dis 2017;4(4):ofx213.

33. Schuetz P, Wirz Y, Sager R, et al. Effect of procalcitonin-guided antibiotic treatment on mortality in acute respiratory infections: a patient level meta-analysis. Lancet Infect Dis 2018;18(1):95–107.

34. Chu DC, Mehta AB, Walkey AJ. Practice patterns and outcomes associated with procalcitonin use in critically ill patients with sepsis. Clin Infect Dis 2017;64(11):1509–15.

35. Messacar K, Parker SK, Todd JK, et al. Implementation of rapid molecular infectious disease diagnostics: the role of diagnostic and antimicrobial stewardship. J Clin Microbiol 2017;55(3):715–23.

36. Dodds Ashley ES, Kaye KS, DePestel DD, et al. Antimicrobial stewardship: philosophy versus practice. Clin Infect Dis 2014;59(Suppl 3):S112–21.

37. DiazGranados CA. Prospective audit for antimicrobial stewardship in intensive care: impact on resistance and clinical outcomes. Am J Infect Control 2012;40(6):526–9.

38. Newland JG, Stach LM, De Lurgio SA, et al. Impact of a prospective-audit-with-feedback antimicrobial stewardship program at a children's hospital. J Pediatric Infect Dis Soc 2012;1(3):179–86.

39. Elligsen M, Walker SA, Pinto R, et al. Audit and feedback to reduce broad-spectrum antibiotic use among intensive care unit patients: a controlled interrupted time series analysis. Infect Control Hosp Epidemiol 2012;33(4):354–61.

40. White AC Jr, Atmar RL, Wilson J, et al. Effects of requiring prior authorization for selected antimicrobials: expenditures, susceptibilities, and clinical outcomes. Clin Infect Dis 1997;25(2):230–9.

41. Pakyz AL, Oinonen M, Polk RE. Relationship of carbapenem restriction in 22 university teaching hospitals to carbapenem use and carbapenem-resistant Pseudomonas aeruginosa. Antimicrob Agents Chemother 2009;53(5):1983–6.

42. Rhodes A, Evans LE, Alhazzani W, et al. Surviving sepsis campaign: international guidelines for management of sepsis and septic shock: 2016. Crit Care Med 2017;45(3):486–552.

43. Vincent JL, Bassetti M, Francois B, et al. Advances in antibiotic therapy in the critically ill. Crit Care (London, England) 2016;20(1):133.

44. Freeman CD, Strayer AH. Mega-analysis of meta-analysis: an examination of meta-analysis with an emphasis on once-daily aminoglycoside comparative trials. Pharmacotherapy 1996;16(6):1093–102.

45. Falagas ME, Tansarli GS, Ikawa K, et al. Clinical outcomes with extended or continuous versus short-term intravenous infusion of carbapenems and piperacillin/tazobactam: a systematic review and meta-analysis. Clin Infect Dis 2013; 56(2):272–82.

46. Tamma PD, Putcha N, Suh YD, et al. Does prolonged beta-lactam infusions improve clinical outcomes compared to intermittent infusions? A meta-analysis and systematic review of randomized, controlled trials. BMC Infect Dis 2011; 11:181.

47. Braykov NP, Morgan DJ, Schweizer ML, et al. Assessment of empirical antibiotic therapy optimisation in six hospitals: an observational cohort study. Lancet Infect Dis 2014;14(12):1220–7.

48. Garnacho-Montero J, Gutierrez-Pizarraya A, Escoresca-Ortega A, et al. De-escalation of empirical therapy is associated with lower mortality in patients with severe sepsis and septic shock. Intensive Care Med 2014;40(1):32–40.

49. Kollef MH, Morrow LE, Niederman MS, et al. Clinical characteristics and treatment patterns among patients with ventilator-associated pneumonia. Chest 2006;129(5):1210–8.

50. Lee TC, Frenette C, Jayaraman D, et al. Antibiotic self-stewardship: trainee-led structured antibiotic time-outs to improve antimicrobial use. Ann Intern Med 2014;161(10 Suppl):S53–8.

51. Pulcini C, Defres S, Aggarwal I, et al. Design of a 'day 3 bundle' to improve the reassessment of inpatient empirical antibiotic prescriptions. J Antimicrob Chemother 2008;61(6):1384–8.

52. Pugh R, Grant C, Cooke RP, et al. Short-course versus prolonged-course antibiotic therapy for hospital-acquired pneumonia in critically ill adults. Cochrane Database Syst Rev 2011;(10):CD007577.

53. Chastre J, Wolff M, Fagon JY, et al. Comparison of 8 vs 15 days of antibiotic therapy for ventilator-associated pneumonia in adults: a randomized trial. JAMA 2003;290(19):2588–98.

54. Sandberg T, Skoog G, Hermansson AB, et al. Ciprofloxacin for 7 days versus 14 days in women with acute pyelonephritis: a randomised, open-label and double-blind, placebo-controlled, non-inferiority trial. Lancet (London, England) 2012;380(9840):484–90.

55. Solomkin JS, Mazuski JE, Bradley JS, et al. Diagnosis and management of complicated intra-abdominal infection in adults and children: guidelines by the Surgical Infection Society and the Infectious Diseases Society of America. Clin Infect Dis 2010;50(2):133–64.

56. Dunbar LM, Wunderink RG, Habib MP, et al. High-dose, short-course levofloxacin for community-acquired pneumonia: a new treatment paradigm. Clin Infect Dis 2003;37(6):752–60.

57. Bartlett JG, Gilbert DN, Spellberg B. Seven ways to preserve the miracle of anti-biotics. Clin Infect Dis 2013;56(10):1445–50.
58. Wright GD. Antibiotic resistance in the environment: a link to the clinic? Curr Opin Microbiol 2010;13(5):589–94.
59. Sikkens JJ, van Agtmael MA, Peters EJG, et al. Behavioral approach to appro-priate antimicrobial prescribing in hospitals: the Dutch Unique Method for Antimi-crobial Stewardship (DUMAS) participatory intervention study. JAMA Intern Med 2017;177(8):1130–8.

Antibiotic Stewardship
Strategies to Minimize Antibiotic Resistance While Maximizing Antibiotic Effectiveness

Cheston B. Cunha, MD*, Steven M. Opal, MD

KEYWORDS

- Antibiotic stewardship • Antibiotic resistance • Optimal antimicrobial dosing
- Pharmacokinetic considerations • Pharmacodynamic considerations

KEY POINTS

- The first consideration in antibiotic selection is antibiotic spectrum, which is based on the usual site-related pathogens, for example, lung, biliary tract, or colon.
- Clinicians should avoid overcovering and over treating colonizing organisms in respiratory secretions and the genitourinary tract.
- The most effective resistance prevention strategies is to preferentially select a low resistance potential antibiotic which should be administered in the highest possible dose without toxicity for the shortest duration.
- Most multidrug-resistant organisms resistance in this setting is due to spread within the intensive care unit from colonized patients, and, to a lesser extent, is related to antimicrobial therapy.

OVERVIEW

An important concern of antibiotic stewardship programs is the selection of empiric antibiotic therapy for sepsis in the hospitalized patient.[1–5] Although the definition of sepsis continues to evolve, stewardship programs need to optimize therapy while minimizing resistance.[6–9] Early, empiric, broad-spectrum antibiotic therapy, preferably within the first hour of the recognition of septic shock, is now the recommended treatment of choice.[7] In the septic patient, antibiotic stewardship is concerned with picking

Conflict of Interest: Neither author has any potential conflict to declare with regard to this article.
Division of Infectious Disease, Rhode Island Hospital, The Miriam Hospital, Brown University Alpert School of Medicine, 593 Eddy Street, Physicians Office Building, Suite #328, Providence, RI 02903, USA
* Corresponding author.
E-mail address: ccunha@lifespan.org

the right antibiotic against the most likely, site-related pathogen while minimizing resistance.[10] Maximizing antibiotic effectiveness depends on pharmacokinetic (PK) and pharmacodynamic (PD) considerations. The antibiotic's resistance potential, which is an inherent antibiotic characteristic, is independent of antibiotic class. Within each antibiotic class, there are high resistance potential as well as low resistance potential antibiotics. PK/PD considerations optimize effectiveness and selection of a low resistance potential antibiotic, minimizing the potential for resistance.[11,12] In hospitals where antibiotic resistance among endemic, gram-negative, bacillary microorganisms is common, antibiotic choices are limited and careful selection of the initial antimicrobial regimen in the septic patient is critical.[13]

The mechanism of action and mechanism of inactivation/resistance does not explain why antibiotics in a class have a high or low resistance potential.[14] Even with high volume or prolonged use, antibiotics with a low resistance potential have little or no resistance, for example, ceftriaxone. Among the third-generation cephalosporins, only ceftazidime, a high resistant potential antibiotic, has been associated with *Pseudomonas aeruginosa* resistance, even with modest use. In contrast, other third-generation cephalosporins are low resistance potential antibiotics and have minimal resistance potential, even with high volume use over long periods of time. Beside inherent antibiotic resistance potential, antibiotic dosing, in part, is related to the emergence of resistance.[10]

ANTIBIOTIC RESISTANCE
In Vitro Susceptibility Testing Versus In Vivo Effectiveness

Antibiotic resistance is a complex concept. There is no international agreement on standard breakpoints that define resistant and susceptible pathogens to specific agents.[13,15] Susceptibility testing is based on achievable serum concentrations using the usual recommended doses of antibiotics. Susceptibility testing is used for rapidly growing organisms and, for this reason, susceptibility testing is not done on non–rapidly growing organisms.[15] Susceptibility of isolates cultured from nonbloodstream sites requires interpretation and extrapolation. In vitro susceptibility testing assumes that the antibiotic is being used in the usual dose to treat a bloodstream infection, and that local conditions at the actual site of infection are similar to the blood. The septic patient may be acidotic, but laboratory susceptibility testing is done at pH 7.4. The chemical composition of susceptibility media also affects susceptibility results.[16,17] With some organisms, in vitro susceptibility testing does not predict in vivo clinical effectiveness.[18]

In the clinical setting, local acidosis, poor perfusion, local hypoxia, and cellular debris as found in an abscess cavity can markedly reduce the activity of some antibiotics, for example, aminoglycosides.[19] For difficult to penetrate target tissues, the clinician must extrapolate from achievable serum concentrations to probable target tissue concentrations.[20] Without such extrapolation, unwary clinicians may conclude that, because the susceptibility report indicated susceptible, that the isolate is susceptible to the antibiotic in all body sites, regardless of local factors and local antibiotic concentrations. In general, if an organism reported as susceptible, it is usually susceptible, depending on the organism and clinically achievable concentrations in serum. However, there are important nonblood sites of infection that are difficult to penetrate, and require a PK estimate of antibiotic concentrations at the target tissue/site of infection.[20] Most antibiotics susceptibilities are reported as susceptible or resistant, but some, for example, penicillin and *Streptococcus pneumoniae*, have 3 different susceptibility breakpoints, that is, susceptible, intermediate, and resistant.[21] These breakpoints also differ between *S pneumoniae* isolated from the cerebrospinal fluid versus isolation of the same pathogen from noncerebrospinal fluid sites.[21] Cefepime also has 3 breakpoints for *P aeruginosa*. In such cases, the question is whether to consider the intermediate susceptibilities as susceptible or resistant. In general, if the achievable serum concentration with usual or high dosing exceeds the minimal inhibitory concentration (MIC) of the intermediate or even moderately resistant organism (at the site of infection), then the isolate should be considered as susceptible rather than resistant.[19,21] This point is important, because many physicians regard susceptibility results as absolute and do not take into account differences in antibiotic concentrations in the absence or presence of inflammation/infection in different body sites, for example, cerebrospinal fluid, bone, prostate, or urine.[4]

CLINICALLY RELEVANT TYPES OF RESISTANCE
Natural or Inherent Resistance

Resistance may be classified by mechanism or type of resistance. The mechanism of resistance is beyond the scope of this article and there are excellent reviews on the subject.[22] However, the mechanism of resistance does not explain important differences in resistance potential among classes of antibiotics. Antibiotic resistance may be considered as intrinsic or acquired. Resistance may also be classified within a class or as a cross-resistance between antibiotic classes. Inherent antibiotic resistance refers to the natural resistance of certain organisms, for example, enterococci are intrinsically resistant to cephalosporins, nafcillin demonstrates inherent resistance to *P aeruginosa*, and so on.[19]

Acquired Resistance

The opposite of natural resistance is acquired resistance, which refers to organisms that were formerly sensitive to various antibiotics but have become resistant. Acquired resistance may be high-level/absolute or relative resistance. High-level/absolute resistance cannot be overcome by increasing antibiotic dosage, that is, resistance is independent of serum concentrations. With high-level resistance, an alternate antibiotic that is effective against the organism should be selected.[23] Similarly, acquired high-level resistance is, for example, gentamicin with *P aeruginosa* isolated with an MIC of greater than 4000 µg/mL and the infection should be treated with another susceptible antibiotic class. Acquired relative resistance affords the clinician an opportunity to apply PK principles to treat the infections at different body sites. These estimates are based on PK principles; data are limited or not available for each individual patient treatment decision.

Class Resistance

Resistance may also be considered within an antibiotic class. For example, *P aeruginosa* resistance to ciprofloxacin may also be resistant to levofloxacin. This is a commonly recognized clinical reality but there are important exceptions, for example, aminoglycosides. For example, *P aeruginosa* not uncommonly is resistant to gentamicin and tobramycin, but susceptible to amikacin. Gentamicin and tobramycin have 6 loci in their structure that are susceptible to aminoglycoside inactivating enzymes that mediate clinical resistance. In contrast, amikacin has only one such locus. For this reason, amikacin is the aminoglycoside most likely to be susceptible with gentamicin and tobramycin resistance with *P aeruginosa*.[19]

Cross-Resistance

In contrast, cross-resistance refers to antibiotic resistance between classes. For reasons that are not entirely clear, an antibiotic can induce resistance in another antibiotic class with 1 or more organisms manifested by an increase in MICs, that is, MIC drift. These problems are often related to permeability mutants or the presence of nonspecific efflux pumps that expel multiple classes of antibiotics out of the cell. For example, with *P aeruginosa*, the use of ciprofloxacin may induce MIC drift that affects other antipseudomonal drugs within the same class, for example, levofloxacin, as well as from other antibiotic classes such as imipenem and ceftazidime. The same is true for other antipseudomonal high resistance potential antibiotics. If imipenem is the primary hospital carbapenem, then MIC creep may be seen with other carbapenems, for example, meropenem and doripenem, as well as other antipseudomonal antibiotics in other classes, such as ciprofloxacin, levofloxacin, gentamicin, and ceftazidime.[23,24] For this reason, if an institution has a resistance problem with a particular organism, such as *P aeruginosa*, a single substitution in formulary from a high resistance potential antibiotic to a low resistance potential antibiotic will not solve the problem. For better control of a *P aeruginosa* resistance problem, all antipseudomonal antibiotics on formulary should be of the low resistance potential variety.[23]

Resistance Potential

Antibiotics can be classified has having a high resistance potential or a low resistance potential. Historically, a low resistance potential antibiotic may be defined as one that has little propensity for the development of resistance, regardless of the volume and duration of use, for example, doxycycline, minocycline, amikacin, or cefepime. In contrast, high resistance antibiotics are likely to be associated with resistance problems, even with limited volume of use. It is not known why, within antibiotic classes, there are both high and low resistance potential antibiotics. Some members of each antibiotic class have not caused resistance, whereas others have been associated with resistance.[24] The third-generation cephalosporin, ceftriaxone, is an example of a low resistance potential antibiotic that, even after decades of high-volume use, shows very little clinically significant resistance with ceftriaxone or other third-generation cephalosporins (with the exception of ceftazidime). Ceftazidime, among the third-generation cephalosporins, is the only high resistance potential antibiotic associated with *P aeruginosa* resistance. Among the fluoroquinolones, ciprofloxacin is the high resistance potential quinolone, whereas levofloxacin and moxifloxacin are low resistance potential antibiotics[23] (**Table 1**).

The message for clinicians is clear. The primary way to prevent resistance is to preferentially use low resistance potential antibiotics instead of high resistance potential antibiotics for any given infection. Almost always, there are other alternatives within the same class of antibiotics that provide the same or better activity against the pathogen than high resistance potential antibiotics.[23,24] Although PD considerations may minimize the resistance potential of high resistance potential antibiotics, the best approach is to preferentially use low resistance potential antibiotics. Resistance may occur if applied in the wrong clinical context, for example, even a low resistance potential antibiotic used to treat an abscess, where concentrations within the abscess are low may predispose to resistance.[25] Intermittently active pathogens living in a biofilm along the surface of a foreign body create an ideal environment for resistance to occur. In situations where there is impaired blood supply or poor tissue penetration problems, resistance may occur with any antibiotic, but certainly are more frequently with high resistance potential antibiotics.[26] In a further effort to limit resistance, treat

Table 1
The inherent resistance potential of selected antibiotics

High Resistance Potential Antibiotics	Usual Resistant Organisms for Each Antibiotic	Preferred Low Resistance Potential Antibiotic Alternatives
Aminoglycosides		
Gentamicin/tobramycin	Pseudomonas aeruginosa	Amikacin
Cephalosporins		
Ceftazidime	P aeruginosa	Cefepime
Tetracyclines		
Tetracycline	Streptococcus pneumoniae Staphylococcus aureus	Doxycycline or minocycline
Quinolones		
Ciprofloxacin	S pneumoniae P aeruginosa	Levofloxacin or moxifloxacin Levofloxacin
Glycopeptides		
Vancomycin	MSSA MRSA	Linezolid or daptomycin or minocycline
Carbapenems		
Imipenem	P aeruginosa	Meropenem or doripenem
Macrolides		
Azithromycin	S pneumoniae	No other macrolide; alternatives include doxycycline, levofloxacin, or moxifloxacin
Dihydrofolate reductase inhibitors		
TMP-SMX	S pneumoniae	Doxycycline

Abbreviations: MRSA, methicillin-resistant *Staphylococcus aureus*; MSSA, methicillin-sensitive *S aureus*; TMP-SMX, trimethoprim-sulfamethoxazole.
Data from Cunha BA. Effective antibiotic-resistance control strategies. Lancet 2001;357(9265):1307–8; and Cunha BA, editor. Antibiotic essentials. 12th edition. Sudbury (MA): Jones & Bartlett Learning; 2013.

for the shortest duration of therapy that eradicates the infection. Longer courses are not more efficacious and may predispose to resistance.[27]

Antibiotic Dosing Consideration to Minimize Resistance and Optimize Effectiveness

PK refers to the concentration and distribution of antibiotics in serum and body fluids as a function of time. Serum concentrations are related peak serum concentrations, serum half-life, protein findings, and renal and hepatic functions. The tissue penetration characteristics of antibiotics are determined by PK parameters, for example, peak serum concentration, protein binding, and volume of distribution.[28–32] Reevaluate the patient for clinical improvement on day 3. If clinical improvement occurs, complete therapy with the same drug.

PD in the treatment of infection refers to antibiotic killing and is described as being either demonstrating concentration-dependent killing, time-dependent killing, or a combination of both. Concentration-dependent killing kinetics refers to the increase in bacterial killing that occurs as antibiotic concentrations are increased above the MIC, and is expressed as serum antibiotic concentration (C_{max}) to the MIC ratio

(C_{max}:MIC).[29,32] Antibiotics that display concentration-dependent killing, such as aminoglycosides, daptomycin, and metronidazole, often demonstrate a postantibiotic effect (PAE), indicating that regrowth of the pathogen is delayed by several hours after adequate blood levels of the antibiotic have disappeared. Antibiotics that display time-dependent killing kinetics are those in which an increase in serum levels does not result in increased killing above the 4 to 5 times MIC of the organism, and are expressed as time of drug concentration above the MIC for the dosing period (T > MIC), for example, β-lactam antibiotics, carbapenems, macrolides.[29] Other antibiotics (eg, fluoroquinolones) express killing kinetics best described by the PD parameter known as area under the concentration time curve over a 24-hour period, that is, area under the curve (AUC_{0-24}:MIC).[30–32]

Interestingly, some antibiotics display both time- and concentration-dependent killing kinetics, for example, doxycycline and vancomycin.[33] Time-dependent killing kinetics does describe the PD of vancomycin with gram-positive cocci with an MIC of less than 1 μg/mL; however, with an MIC of greater than 1 μg/mL, vancomycin displays concentration-depending killing kinetics. Even with antibiotics that demonstrate time-dependent killing, there is no downside in using high-dose antimicrobial therapy.[34]

In general, bacteriostatic antibiotics display time-dependent killing kinetics, whereas bactericidal antibiotics demonstrate concentration-dependent killing kinetics and some antibiotics exhibit both types of killing kinetics. Doxycycline, for example, which displays time-dependent killing kinetics, is bactericidal against some pathogens at high concentrations, that is, concentration-dependent killing kinetics.[33] Penicillins, monobactams, and carbapenems display time-dependent killing kinetics, but are bactericidal[35] (**Tables 2** and **3**).

Table 2
Antibiotic dosing: PK/PD considerations[a]

Antibiotic PK/PD Parameters	Optimal Dosing Strategies
Concentration-dependent antibiotics (C_{max}: MIC) • Quinolones • Aminoglycosides • Vancomycin if MIC ≥1 μg/mL • Doxycycline • Tigecycline • Colistin	Use highest effective dose (without toxicity)
Time-dependent antibiotics (T > MIC) • PCN concentrations > MIC for 60% of the dosing interval • β-Lactam concentrations > MIC for 75% of the dosing interval • Carbapenems concentrations > MIC for 40% of the dosing interval • Vancomycin if MIC ≤1 μg/mL	Use high doses (which increase serum concentrations and also increases T > MIC for more of the dosing interval)

Other antibiotics (C_{max}: MIC/T > MIC and/or AUC_{0-24}/MIC)
• Quinolones
  ○ >125 (effective)
  ○ >250 (more effective)
	Use highest effective dose (without toxicity)

Abbreviations: AUC, area under the curve; C_{max}, peak serum concentrations; MIC, minimal inhibitory concentration; PD, pharmacodynamic; PK, pharmacokinetic.
[a] Depends on log phase of bacteria, site of infection, inoculation size and post antibiotic effect (PAE).
Data from Refs.[29,36,40]

Table 3
Antibiotics: relevant pharmacokinetic characteristics in the ICU

Antibiotic PK Parameters	Sepsis ↑ with Capillary Permeability[a]	Suggested Dosing Recommendations[b]
Water-soluble antibiotics (low V_d water soluble) • Renally eliminated • High serum concentrations • Limited tissue penetration	• ↑ V_d → ↓ serum concentrations	• ↑ Dose of hydrophilic antibiotic • Change to a lipid soluble antibiotic
Lipid-soluble antibiotics (high V_d → lipid soluble) • Hepatically eliminated • High tissue penetration • Good serum concentrations		• No change in V_d → No change in serum or tissue concentrations • No Change needed

Abbreviations: ICU, intensive care unit; V_d, volume of distribution.
[a] Also with mechanical ventilation, burns, and hypoalbuminemia. Intravascular → interstitial fluid shifts and sustained high cardiac output with increased renal clearance.
[b] Use maximum tolerated, initial dosing strategies.
Data from Roberts JA, Lipman J. Pharmacokinetic issues for antibiotics in the critically ill patient. Crit Care Med 2009;37(3):840–51.

Quinolones

Quinolones primarily display concentration-dependent killing kinetics, but also display some time-dependent killing kinetic characteristics as well. The AUC_{0-24}:MIC ratios have been shown to correlate with clinical outcomes, that is, an AUC_{0-24}:MIC ratio of greater than 125 is usually considered predictive of efficacy in gram-negative infections. However, a high AUC_{0-24}:MIC ratio of greater than 250 may be optimal and may reduce resistance.[36] Taking these factors into account, quinolone dosing should be optimized to use the highest possible dose while avoiding toxicity, which optimizes not only the C_{max}:MIC, but also AUC_{0-24}:MIC ratio to minimize the potential for the emergence of resistant mutants.[37–39]

Vancomycin

PD descriptions of vancomycin differ depending on staphylococcal MICs. With MICs of greater than 1, vancomycin exhibits concentration-dependent killing kinetics, whereas with MICs of less than 1, time-dependent killing kinetics describes vancomycin's action. In addition, vancomycin use can result in an increase in staphylococcal cell wall thickness, which results in decreased permeability of vancomycin, as well as other antibiotics, into the organism. This permeability-mediated resistance is manifested either by an increase in MICs to vancomycin as well as other gram-positive organisms.[34] Patients with osteomyelitis can be treated for months without adverse effects and optimal outcomes with high-dose vancomycin. Because current formulations of vancomycin are essentially nonnephrotoxic, the use of high-dose vancomycin is preferred. Giving high-dose vancomycin, for example, 60 mg/kg (intravenously [IV]) every 24 hours or 2 g (IV) every 12 hours is a reasonable strategy in adults with normal kidney function, because this may optimize efficacy and minimize resistance.[19] As with other antibiotics, low-dose vancomycin has been associated with the development of resistance.

β-Lactams

β-Lactams display time-dependent killing kinetics, and optimal killing occurs when antibiotic concentrations are approximately 5 times the MIC of the organism. Above

5 times the MIC of the organism, there is no additional killing.[36,40] As long as the serum concentrations remain above the MIC for greater than 75% of the dosing interval, susceptible organisms are inhibited. β-Lactams are bactericidal and, although they have a short PAE with gram-positive bacteria, they have no appreciable PAE with gram-negative organisms. Because β-lactams demonstrate a time-dependent killing kinetics, some investigators have advocated more frequent dosing or continuous infusion to maintain effective concentration throughout the dosing period.[41–43] For most hospitals, a preferred strategy is to either increase the dose duration or shorten the dosing interval. Higher dosing also results in higher serum concentrations over most of the dosing period.[36] Therefore, a high dose with a prolonged dosing duration (2–3 hours) is an optimal way administer β-lactam antibiotics, particularly in the intensive care setting, for maximum effectiveness and minimal resistance potential.[36,40] From a tissue penetration perspective, higher serum levels are preferable with time-dependent antibiotics, for example, β-lactams. Higher doses mean higher tissue levels, because tissue penetration is a percentage of peak serum concentration; with time- and concentration-dependent antibiotics, the higher the serum concentration, the higher the target tissue levels.[19]

Carbapenems

Carbapenems resemble β-lactams structurally and have similar PD characteristics to other β-lactams but differ in their allergic potential. Carbapenem serum concentrations should be more than 5 times the MIC.[40] Carbapenems serum concentrations should be maintained for at least 40% of the dosing interval in contrast with penicillins (~60%) and cephalosporins (~75%). The resistance potential of carbapenems seems to be not only related to PD parameters, but also to the inherent resistance potential of the antibiotic; for example, imipenem has a high resistance potential, whereas meropenem and doripenem have a low resistance potential.[19,23] Again, the best strategy seems to be to use high-dose carbapenems to optimize effectiveness and not only related to PD parameters.[36,40,44,45]

Daptomycin

Daptomycin is bactericidal against gram-positive organisms, displays concentration-dependent kinetics, and has a prolonged PAE (>6 hours). As with other antibiotics, daptomycin displays dual PD characteristics, that is, C_{max}/MIC as well as AUC_{0-24}:MIC. Recommended dosing regimens for daptomycin are related to the site of infection, that is, 4 mg/kg (IV) every 24 hours for skin and soft tissue infections or 6 mg/kg (IV) every 24 hours for bacteremia.[19] For relatively resistant organisms, high-dose daptomycin 10 to 12 mg/kg (IV) every 24 hours has been used successfully, using various regimens; as with other antibiotics, low doses predispose to resistance.[46] Daptomycin is approximately half as active against group D streptococci as staphylococci. It is not surprising that the usual dose may result in enterococcal resistance with vancomycin-sensitive and well as vancomycin-resistant enterococci.[47]

Linezolid

Linezolid displays time-dependent killing kinetics and is bacteriostatic against staphylococci and enterococci, but it is bactericidal against non–group D streptococci. Linezolid has been used successful in treating acute bacterial endocarditis, where bactericidal antibiotics are theoretically preferred. The outcomes of therapy with linezolid for *Staphylococcus aureus* acute bacterial endocarditis is comparable with therapy using bactericidal antistaphylococcal antibiotics.[19] Prolonged linezolid therapy

Table 4
Empiric antibiotic coverage for common infections in the ICU

Infection Type/ Site	Usual Pathogen at Site	Usual Nonpathogens at Site	Preferred Empiric Therapy with Low Resistance Potential Antibiotics	Penicillin Allergy
CVC-associated bacteremia[a]	MSSA MRSA CoNS GNBs (aerobic) VSE	Bacteroides fragilis Non–group D streptococci	Meropenem plus either vancomycin (if MRSA likely) or linezolid (if VRE likely)	Meropenem plus either vancomycin (if MRSA likely) or linezolid (if VRE likely)
Intraabdominal sepsis				
Cholecystitis/ cholangitis	Escherichia coli Klebsiella pneumoniae VSE	B fragilis	Levofloxacin or moxifloxacin	Levofloxacin or moxifloxacin
Peritonitis/ colon perforation	B fragilis GNBs (aerobic)	Non–group D streptococci	Ertapenem or piperacillin/ tazobactam or moxifloxacin or tigecycline	Ertapenem or moxifloxacin or tigecycline
VAP/NP	Pseudomonas aeruginosa GNBs (aerobic)	B fragilis MSSA/MRSA VSE/VRE Burkholderia cepacia Acinetobacter baumannii Stenotrophomonas maltophilia	Meropenem or doripenem or levofloxacin (750 mg) or cefepime	Meropenem or doripenem or levofloxacin (750 mg)
Urosepsis				
Community acquired	GNBs (aerobic) VSE	B fragilis MSSA/MRSA	Piperacillin/ tazobactam or meropenem	Meropenem
Nosocomial	P aeruginosa GNBs (aerobic)	B fragilis MSSA/MRSA	Piperacillin/ tazobactam or meropenem	Meropenem
Skin and soft tissue infections				
Cellulitis	Group A, B, C, and G streptococci	MSSA/MRSA	Ceftriaxone or cefazolin	Vancomycin or clindamycin
Abscess	MSSA/MRSA	Group A, B, C, and G streptococci	Ceftaroline or minocycline or vancomycin or linezolid	Vancomycin or linezolid or minocycline

Abbreviations: CoNS, coagulase negative staphylococci; CVC, central venous catheter; GNB, gram-negative bacilli; ICU, intensive care unit; MRSA, methicillin resistant S aureus; MSSA, methicillin sensitive S aureus; VAP/NP, ventilator-associated pneumonia/nosocomial pneumonia; VRE, vancomycin resistant enterococci; VSE, vancomycin sensitive enterococci.
  [a] Remove/replace CVC ASAP.
  From Cunha CB, Cunha BA, editors. Antibiotic essentials. 15th edition. New Delhi: Jaypee Brothers Medical Publishers Pvt. Ltd; 2017; with permission.

has been shown to be associated with resistance, as has been the case with daptomycin.

Tigecycline

Because tigecycline is a derivative of tetracycline, tigecycline is considered to display time-dependent killing characteristics, but the optimal dosing regimen for tigecycline is yet to be determined. Tigecycline requires a loading dose, because it has a high volume of distribution, that is, 8 L/kg, to achieve therapeutic serum concentrations. Because tigecycline is generally well-tolerated, a higher than the usual loading dose of 100 mg, that is, 200 to 400 mg, may be necessary for relatively resistant gram-negative organisms.[48,49] The recommended tigecycline maintenance dose is 50 mg (IV) every 12 hours. Because the half-life of tigecycline is so long (half-life of 42 hours), it makes no sense to administer a drug with such a long half-life every 12 hours. Pharmacokinetically, after the initial loading dose tigecycline, the maintenance dose (one-half of the loading dose) should be dosed every 24 hours and not by split dose.[15] The concern about the potential therapeutic failures of tigecycline in the literature relate to treating organism innately tigecycline-resistant, for example, *P aeruginosa,* or to underdosing.

SUMMARY

the key elements in this article may be summarized by the following principle: use high-dose, low resistance potential antibiotics for the shortest duration to achieve clinical elimination of the infection. The first antibiotic dose is critical and care should be taken to ensure adequate levels in blood and tissues to inhibit the infecting microorganism and limit resistance potential. Use adjunctive measures when necessary, that is, drainage of abscesses, or relief of obstruction, or removal of infected devices. Use the highest dose of an antibiotic, without toxicity, where there is likely relative resistance. Avoid the temptation to initiate treatment for isolates cultured from colonized sites. Colonizing organisms are more difficult to eradicate than infection, and treatment of colonization is often prolonged. This is a common source of in vivo development of antibiotic resistance by already relatively resistant organisms.[4] Empiric antibiotic therapy should not be used to treat otherwise unexplained fever and leukocytosis or noninfectious mimics of infections. Unnecessary therapy is expensive and may result in potential drug side effects, *C difficile,* or increased antimicrobial resistance.[50]

In selecting an empiric antibiotic for the patient with sepsis, clinicians should consider spectrum (appropriate for infection site), degree of activity against the site-related pathogen (having demonstrated clinical effectiveness), and resistance potential. When possible, select a low resistance potential antibiotic with the correct spectrum and a high degree of activity against the pathogen. Make every effort to optimize dosing based on PK/PD considerations (use the highest, nontoxic, tolerated dose), and treat for the shortest duration that eradicates the infection (**Table 4**).

REFERENCES

1. Cunha CB, Varughese CA, Mylonakis E. Antimicrobial stewardship programs (ASPs): the devil is in the details. Virulence 2013;4:147–9.

2. Hurford A, Morris AM, Fisman DN, et al. Linking antimicrobial prescribing to antimicrobial resistance in the ICU: before and after an antimicrobial stewardship program. Epidemics 2012;4:203–10.

3. Rimawi RH, Mazer MA, Siraj DS, et al. Impact of regular collaboration between infectious diseases and critical care practitioners on antimicrobial utilization and patient outcome. Crit Care Med 2013;41:2099–107.
4. Njoku JA, Hermsen ED. Antimicrobial stewardship in the intensive care unit: a focus of potential pitfalls. J Pharm Pract 2010;23:50–60.
5. Amer MR, Akhras NS, Mahmood WA, et al. Antimicrobial stewardship program implementation in a medical intensive care unit at a tertiary care hospital in Saudi Arabia. Ann Saudi Med 2013;33:547–54.
6. Vincent JL, Opal SM, Marshall JC, et al. Sepsis definitions: time for change. Lancet 2013;381:774–5.
7. Singer M, Deutschman CS, Seymour CW, et al. The third international consensus definitions for sepsis and septic shock (Sepsis-3). JAMA 2016;315(8):801–10.
8. Erdem H, Inan A, Altindis S, et al. Surveillance, control and management of infections in intensive care units in Southern Europe, Turkey and Iran—a prospective multicenter point prevalence study. J Infect 2014;68:131–40.
9. Frakking FN, Rottier WC, Dorigo-Zetsma JW, et al. Appropriateness of empirical treatment and outcome in bacteremia caused by extended-spectrum-β-lactamase-producing bacteria. Antimicrob Agents Chemother 2013;57:3092–9.
10. Martinex MN, Papich MG, Drusano GL. Dosing regimen matters: the importance of early intervention and rapid attainment of the pharmacokinetic/pharmacodynamic target. Antimicrob Agents Chemother 2012;56:2795–805.
11. Papadimitriou-Oliveris M, Marangos M, Fligou F, et al. KPC- producing Klebsiella pneumoniae enteric colonization acquired during intensive care unit stay: the significance of risk factors for its development and its impact on mortality. Diagn Microbiol Infect Dis 2013;77:169–73.
12. Pogue JM, Marchaim D, Kaye D, et al. Revisiting "older" antimicrobials in the era of multidrug resistance. Pharmacotherapy 2011;31:912–21.
13. Kahlmeter G. Defining antibiotic resistance-towards international harmonization. Ups J Med Sci 2014;119:78–86.
14. Baquero F, Coque TM, Canton R. Counteracting antibiotic resistance: breaking barriers among antibacterial strategies. Expert Opin Ther Targets 2014;31:1–11.
15. Turnidge J, Paterson DL. Setting and revising antibacterial susceptibility breakpoints. Clin Microbiol Infect 2007;20:391–408.
16. Domenico P, O'Leary R, Cunha BA. Differential effects of bismuth and salicylate salts on the antibiotic susceptibility of Pseudomonas aeruginosa. Eur J Clin Microbiol Infect Dis 1992;11:170–5.
17. Cunha BA. Problems arising in antimicrobial therapy due to false susceptibility testing. J Chemother 1997;1:25–35.
18. Cunha BA. Minocycline versus doxycycline for methicillin-resistant Staphylococcus aureus (MRSA): in vitro susceptibility versus in vivo effectiveness. Int J Antimicrob Agents 2010;35:517–8.
19. Cunha BA, editor. Antibiotic essentials. 12th edition. Sudbury (MA): Jones & Bartlett; 2013.
20. Lodise TP, Butterfield J. Use of pharmacodynamic principles to inform β-lactam dosing: "S" does not always mean success. J Hosp Med 2011;6:S16–23.
21. Cunha BA. Clinical relevance of penicillin-resistant Streptococcus pneumoniae. Semin Respir Infect 2002;17:204–14.
22. Pop-Vicas A, Opal SM. The Clinical impact of multidrug-resistant gram-negative bacilli in the management of septic shock. Virulence 2014;5:206–12.
23. Cunha BA. Antibiotic resistance: effective control strategies. Lancet 2001;357: 1307–8, 1101.

24. Cunha BA. Strategies to control antibiotic resistance. Semin Resp Infect 2000;21: 3–8.
25. Cunha BA. Antibiotic tissue penetration. Bull N Y Acad Med 1983;59:443–9.
26. Cunha BA. Antibiotic resistance control in the CCU. In: Cunha BA, editor. Infectious diseases in critical care medicine. 2nd edition. New York: Informa Healthcare; 2007. p. 609–24.
27. Opal SM. ACP journal club. Review: short-course antibiotics in hospital-acquired pneumonia do not affect mortality. Ann Intern Med 2012;156:JC3–13.
28. Ambrose PG, Owens RC Jr, Quintiliani R, et al. Antibiotic use in the critical care unit. Crit Care Clin 1998;14:283–308.
29. Roberts JA, Lipman J. Pharmacokinetic issues for antibiotics in the critically ill patient. Crit Care Med 2009;37(3):840–51.
30. Owens RC Jr, Shorr AF. Rational dosing of antimicrobial agents: pharmacokinetic and pharmacodynamic strategies. Am J Health Syst Pharm 2009;66:S23–30.
31. Winterboer TM, Lecci KA, Olsen KM. Continuing education: alternative approaches to optimizing antimicrobial pharmacodynamics in critically ill patients. J Pharm Pract 2010;23:6–18.
32. Drusano GL. Antimicrobial pharmacodynamics: critical interactions of "bug and drug." Nat Rev Microbiol 2004;2:289–300.
33. Cunha BA, Domenico P, Cunha CB. Pharmacodynamics of doxycycline. Clin Microbiol Infect 2000;6:270–3.
34. Cunha BA. Vancomycin revisited: a reappraisal of clinical use. Crit Care Clin 2008;24:393–420.
35. Goff DA, Nicolau DP. When pharmacodynamics trump costs: an antimicrobial stewardship program's approach to selecting optimal antimicrobial agents. Clin Ther 2013;35:766–71.
36. Roberts JA, Pharm B, Kruger P, et al. Antibiotic resistance – what's dosing got to do with it? Crit Care Med 2008;36:2433–40.
37. Noreddin AM, Elkhatib WF. Levofloxacin in the treatment of community-acquired pneumonia. Expert Rev Anti Infect Ther 2010;8:505–14.
38. Gous A, Lipman J, Scibante J, et al. Fluid shifts have no influence on ciprofloxacin pharmacokinetics in intensive care patients with intra-abdominal sepsis. Int J Antimicrob Agents 2005;26:50–5.
39. Zelenitsky SA, Ariano RE. Support for higher ciprofloxacin AUC24/MIC targets in treating Enterobacteriaceae bloodstream infection. J Antimicrob Chemother 2010;65:1725–32.
40. Roberts JA, Lipman J. Optimizing use of beta-lactam antibiotics in the critically ill. Semin Respir Crit Care Med 2007;28:579–85.
41. McKinnon PS, Paladine JA, Schentag JJ. Evaluation of area under the inhibitory curve (AUIC) and time above the minimum inhibitory concentration (T>MIC) as predictors of outcome for cefepime and ceftazidime in serious bacterial infections. Int J Antimicrob Agents 2008;31:345–51.
42. Roberts JA, Paratz J, Paratz E, et al. Continuous infusion of beta lactam antibiotics in severe infections: a review of its role. Int J Antimicrob Agents 2007;30: 111–8.
43. Roberts JA, Boots R, Rickard CM, et al. Is continuous infusion ceftriaxone better than once-a- day dosing in intensive care? A randomized controlled pilot study. J Antimicrob Chemother 2006;59:285–91.
44. Ogutlu A, Guclu E, Karabay O, et al. Effects of Carbapenem consumption on the prevalence of Acinetobacter infection in intensive care unit patients. Ann Clin Microbiol Antimicrob 2014;13:7.

45. Palmore TN, Henderson DK. Carbapenem-resistant Enterobacteriaceae: a call for cultural change. Ann Int Med 2014;160:567–70.

46. Cunha BA, Eisenstein LE, Hamid NS. Pacemaker-induced Staphylococcus aureus mitral valve acute bacterial endocarditis complicated by persistent bacteremia from a coronary stent: cure with prolonged/high-dose daptomycin without toxicity. Heart Lung 2006;35:207–11.

47. Cunha BA, Mickail N, Eisenstein L. E. faecalis vancomycin-sensitive enterococcal bacteremia unresponsive to a vancomycin tolerant strain successfully treated with high-dose daptomycin. Heart & Lung 2007;36:456–61.

48. Cunha BA. Once-daily tigecycline therapy of multidrug-resistant and non-multidrug-resistant gram-negative bacteremias. J Chemother 2007;19:232–3.

49. Cunha BA. Pharmacokinetic considerations regarding tigecycline for multidrug-resistant (MDR) Klebsiella pneumoniae or MDR Acinetobacter baumannii urosepsis. J Clin Microbiol 2009;47:1613.

50. Shoai Tehrani M, Hajage D, Fihman V, et al. Gram-negative bacteremia: which empirical antibiotic therapy? Med Mal Infect 2014;44:159–66.

Creative Collaborations in Antimicrobial Stewardship

Using the Centers for Disease Control and Prevention's Core Elements as Your Guide

Priya Nori, MD[a],*, Yi Guo, PharmD[a], Belinda Ostrowsky, MD, MPH[b]

KEYWORDS

- Antimicrobial stewardship programs • Quality collaboratives • Multidisciplinary
- Core elements of stewardship

KEY POINTS

- Antimicrobial stewardship programs (ASPs) are built on a foundation of collaboration across multiple disciplines within the health system infrastructure and with external partners.
- Daily collaborations with pharmacy, microbiology, clinical services, and infection prevention are core activities of stewardship.
- Key stakeholders in ASP success and sustainability include health system executives, departmental and divisional leaders, patient safety and quality, postgraduate training programs, medical schools, and other health professionals.
- ASPs should strive to participate in regional and national quality collaboratives to help advance their agendas, adapt successful interventions from other institutions and establish stewardship benchmarks and best practices. Collaboratives can also assist stewardship programs meet the challenges of impending regulatory requirements.
- Collaboration with neighboring stewardship programs and public health agencies can result in successful innovations in policy, education, scholarship, quality improvement and research.

INTRODUCTION

A 2007 *Harvard Business Review* article entitled "Eight Ways to Build Collaborative Teams"[1] suggests that successful collaborators encourage communication, model

Authors have no commercial or financial conflicts of interest or funding sources for this activity.
[a] Antimicrobial Stewardship Program, Montefiore Health System, Albert Einstein College of Medicine, 111 East 210th Street, Bronx, NY 10467, USA; [b] Antimicrobial Stewardship & Hospital Epidemiology, Antimicrobial Stewardship Program, Montefiore Health System, Albert Einstein College of Medicine, 111 East 210th Street, Bronx, NY 10467, USA
* Corresponding author. Montefiore Medical Center, 3411 Wayne Avenue, # 4H, Bronx, NY 10467.
E-mail address: pnori@montefiore.org

collaborative behavior, mentor and coach other to build networks across boundaries, ensure team building as a requisite skill, and foster a strong sense of community among team members (**Table 1**).[1] These attributes pave the way for success in myriad settings, including antimicrobial stewardship.

Successful antimicrobial stewardship programs (ASPs) harness the diverse expertise of physicians, pharmacists, nurses, microbiologists, and infection preventionists.[2] Unique opportunities for stewardship collaboration exist in daily exchanges with colleagues, challenging clinical cases from the wards, hospital patient safety initiatives, or exciting new research presented at professional society meetings. The following scenario is an illustrative example of a multidisciplinary collaborative to implement a stewardship and quality improvement initiative with a high potential impact on the hospital.

Antimicrobial stewardship vignette 1

At a recent Infectious Diseases Society of America (IDSA) conference, you attended a research presentation on the procalcitonin (PCT) assay as a biomarker of bacterial infection used to prevent unnecessary antibiotic use when coupled with antimicrobial stewardship. The presenter, the stewardship pharmacists at a neighboring facility in New York City, touted several important outcomes of a stewardship-guided PCT algorithm at his facility, namely, reduced days of antibiotic therapy, reduced length of stay and readmissions, and lack of adverse outcomes.[3] You are intrigued by its potential value as stewardship tool at your own institution, which has not yet adopted this test despite approval from the Food and Drug Administration (FDA) for lower respiratory tract infection and sepsis in February 2017.[4] You ask your infectious diseases (ID) fellow to present a review of the latest PCT literature at your ID divisional grand rounds.[5] You invite several important stakeholders to the presentation, including the director of clinical pathology, the director of the emergency department (ED), and the director of quality improvement. After a very thoughtful discussion, a decision is made to pilot the PCT assay for lower respiratory tract infection in the ED. A multidisciplinary task force of experts (stewardship, ID, pulmonology, pathology, quality, information technology, and emergency medicine) is assembled. You invite the IDSA speaker to present his research and serve as an expert consultant to the task force. Over the next 12 months, the PCT initiative is implemented at your facility and the multidisciplinary task force studies its impact on antibiotic utilization, length of stay, mortality, *Clostridium difficile* incidence, and readmissions. The findings are submitted for publication to a reputable journal.

As antimicrobial stewards in New York City (NYC), the authors' goal is to personalize antimicrobial management to their complex patient population, prescribers, and multidrug-resistant pathogens of their local ecosystem. In 2008, the Montefiore Health System established an interdisciplinary ASP to meet the demands of the authors' academic medical center in the Bronx, New York, a heavily resource-limited setting within NYC. The program is co-led by physicians and clinical pharmacists certified in ID and antimicrobial stewardship. The ASP directors oversee stewardship operations at 3 campuses and a pediatric hospital (inclusive of more than 1400 beds in all). The Montefiore ASP recently implemented an ambulatory stewardship program with support from the United Hospital Fund, a local health care policy and research organization. The Centers for Disease Control and Prevention's (CDC) core elements of stewardship have served as the framework for the authors' ASP charter and strategic plan.[6] The backbone of the authors' program is a tiered, upfront restriction policy and robust prescriber educational curriculum.[7] This component is supplemented by numerous pharmacy-driven actions and systematic audit and feedback to prescribers.

The IDSA and the Society for Healthcare Epidemiology of America (SHEA) describe several necessary structural components of a successful ASP and state that

Table 1	
Eight attributes of effective collaborators	
Attribute	**Description**
1. Invest in signature relationship practices.	Create an environment that demonstrates a commitment to collaboration.
2. Model collaborative behavior.	Teams collaborate better when behavior is modeled by executives.
3. Create a gift culture.	Provide mentoring and coaching and help others build networks across boundaries.
4. Ensure the requisite skills.	The skills include relationship building, communication, and conflict resolution.
5. Support a strong sense of community.	It enhances comfort and knowledge sharing.
6. Assign effective team leaders.	Team leaders should be both task and relationship oriented.
7. Build on heritage relationships.	Assemble a team in which several members already know each other.
8. Understand role clarity and task ambiguity.	Cooperation increases when the roles are well defined yet the team has freedom to achieve the task.

Adapted from Gratton L, Erickson TJ. Eight ways to build collaborative teams. Harvard Business Review. 2007; with permission.

expanding a program's influence on rational antibiotic prescribing is a collaborative effort with leadership and frontline staff.[8] To be recognized and adopted throughout the medical center a stewardship program must

1. Secure investment of resources and ideological support from hospital leadership to promote stewardship.
2. Forge successful relationships with diverse medical and surgical services.
3. Identify stewardship champions to promote rational antibiotic use in the acute care, long-term care, and ambulatory spheres.

Collaboration between stewardship and clinical microbiology colleagues is one of the authors' most fruitful partnerships. The Montefiore ASP interacts with the microbiology laboratory on a daily basis. Together the authors' have developed institutional antibiograms, algorithms for susceptibility testing and cascades for result reporting, *Clostridium difficile* testing algorithms, electronic order entry upgrades to improve reporting and interpretation of microbiology results, and protocols for use of multiplex polymerase chain reaction platforms. The authors have also implemented matrix-assisted laser desorption/ionization time-of-flight mass spectrometry and studied its impact across the medical center.[9,10] Diagnostic stewardship of existing and emerging rapid molecular technology is necessary to educate providers on their optimal use to impact patient care and prevent unnecessary resource utilization.[11] These activities represent a snapshot of the authors' integral relationship with the microbiology laboratory. An article by Dr Emilio Bouza and colleagues' article, "Role of the Clinical Microbiology Laboratory in Antimicrobial Stewardship," in the stewardship issue of *Medical Clinics of North America* addresses ASP and microbiology in more detail.

External partnerships with the local health department and neighboring stewardship programs also provide myriad opportunities for collaboration on policy development, education, and research.[7] Given the recent antibiotic use reporting requirements, collaboration with quality organizations adept at harnessing information technology to extract and organize antibiotic use data may be crucial to help sustain stewardship programs. Through such partnerships, local and multicenter antibiotic use data can be collected and reported to stakeholders to promote rational use.[12]

THE CENTERS FOR DISEASE CONTROL AND PREVENTION'S CORE ELEMENTS OF STEWARDSHIP

Using the CDC's core elements of hospital antibiotic stewardship programs as the scaffold for the remaining article, the authors present illustrative examples of vital multidisciplinary partnerships, which have advanced their mission of promoting rational antibiotic use locally, regionally, and nationally (**Table 2**).

Leadership Commitment

Chief executive, chief medical, quality and safety officers must share the ASP philosophy of improved patient outcomes through judicious antimicrobial prescribing.

Table 2
Important stewardship collaborations within Centers for Disease Control and Prevention's core elements framework

Core Element	Stakeholders	Example
1. Leadership commitment	Health system CEO, CMO, division and department heads of medical and surgical services	Ideological support, allocation of dedicated resources and stewardship efforts, liaisons to external partnerships with reputable quality organizations
2. Accountability	ID/ASP-trained pharmacists and physicians working in concert with shared goals and vision	Physician and pharmacy parallel leadership with diverse skill sets to oversee different aspects of the program, provide mentoring and training of future stewards
3. Drug expertise	Pharmacy, other clinical services, patients	Specialized expertise in antiretroviral drug management lead to a collaborative initiative of ARV stewardship for patients with HIV
4. Action	Patients, prescribers, hospital leaders, patient safety, and quality	CAP quality initiative with ED, transition-of-care OPAT program, (collaborations with leaders in quality and improvement)
5. Tracking 6. Reporting	Prescribers, hospital leaders, ASP members	Regional and national stewardship collaboratives providing benchmark data and enhancing stewardship capabilities
7. Education	Medical students, nurses, postgraduate trainees, attending physicians	Multidisciplinary medical school patient safety seminar; ID fellows' workshop on stewardship, infection prevention, epidemiology, and public health

Abbreviations: ARV, antiretroviral; CAP, community-acquired pneumonia; CEO, chief executive officer; CMO, chief medical officer; HIV, human immunodeficiency virus; OPAT, outpatient parenteral antibiotic therapy.

Adapted from Centers for Disease Control and Prevention (CDC). Core elements of hospital antibiotic stewardship programs. Available at: https://www.cdc.gov/antibiotic-use/healthcare/implementation/core-elements.html. Accessed April 25, 2018.

Ideally, the health system administration understands new accreditation standards concerning antimicrobial stewardship and provides adequate support to either initiate or expand ASP to uphold these standards. C-suite leaders are important influencers of the stewardship, patient safety, and quality agendas at the medical center. Their connections to other health care systems and external quality organizations can open channels to unique collaborations and funding opportunities for stewardship. The Montefiore ASP has developed a long-standing partnership with several regional and national health policy, quality, and research organizations, such as the Greater New York Hospital Association (GNYHA) and the United Hospital Fund (UFH). These relationships were initially forged through Montefiore leadership connections. Montefiore ASP has served as program faculty for successful certificate training programs in acute care and long-term care stewardship sponsored by these organizations. These training seminars address a range of stewardship topics, such as best practices in the management of asymptomatic bacteriuria, C difficile, acute respiratory infections, and skin and soft tissue infections. Participants are provided with audit tools and point prevalence surveys to complete and feedback to providers at their home institutions.

As members of UHF's outpatient stewardship initiative of 24 practices from 8 hospitals in metropolitan NYC, the authors have received funding to pilot ambulatory stewardship interventions aimed at reducing inappropriate antibiotic use for viral respiratory infections.[12] Likewise, as members of the multicenter Partnership for Quality Care, a national organization representing large health care systems and health care worker groups throughout the country, the Montefiore ASP collaborated with 12 US hospital systems to conduct a point prevalence survey of antibiotic use across 47 intensive care units (ICUs) to identify opportunities for focused stewardship intervention. Participating hospitals received aggregate benchmark data on ICU antibiotic use across diverse hospital systems to study and share with the authors' frontline ICU providers,[13] thereby advancing a shared mission of improved patient care.

Accountability

Ideally, physician and pharmacy leaders with the requisite training in stewardship and ID oversee ASPs.[8] Both should possess the credentials, administrative acumen, enthusiasm for educational curriculum development, and a strong desire to train and mentor future stewardship leaders. A firm understanding of microbiologic principles, national and local susceptibility patterns, emerging diagnostics, and other important ID concepts is fundamental to both roles. Physician stewards have experience managing multidisciplinary teams and interface with hospital hospital leaders who can influence behavior change concerning antibiotic prescribing.[2] Stewardship pharmacists possess a deep understanding of pharmacologic principles governing stewardship, approach data with rigor, and are facile with important stewardship reporting metrics.[14] As long as goals and priorities align, diverse skill sets, management, and communication styles should be viewed as an asset to the program. The stewardship physician-pharmacist partnership is at the core of any successful stewardship program. Each of the authors' Montefiore campuses has a complementary team of ID-trained physicians and stewardship pharmacists who work in tandem to address daily and long-term ASP goals.

Drug Expertise

The authors' ASP physicians and pharmacists constantly strive to improve prescribing throughout the health system and introduce formulary revisions to reflect newly published research and guidelines. This endeavor is achieved in collaboration with Montefiore's multidisciplinary Antibiotic Subcommittee of the Pharmacy and Therapeutics

Committee. The following is a novel initiative tailored to the authors' unique Bronx population, which still has high human immunodeficiency virus (HIV) prevalence compared with other counties in New York State.[15] In collaboration with the clinical HIV service at Montefiore, the authors' stewardship pharmacists regularly review new antiretroviral (ARV) agents and adjust their hospital formulary accordingly, removing older more toxic agents and adding newly FDA approved agents. Through audit of inpatient ARV regimens, the authors identified a novel patient safety opportunity and implemented a focused ARV stewardship intervention. Medication reconciliation is performed, and ARV regimens are reviewed for completeness and drug-drug interactions with other agents. The stewardship pharmacist and HIV clinician team adjust doses for fluctuating creatinine clearance. Customized electronic order sets were developed accordingly to prevent ARV prescribing errors and assist inpatient teams select the most appropriate regimens for patients with HIV.[16]

Action

Stewardship actions, such as formulary restrictions, institutional treatment guidelines, syndrome-specific order sets, antibiotic de-escalation timeouts, and intravenous (IV) to oral switches are the central functions of any ASP. These core activities can lay the foundation for larger-scale interventions with a potentially high impact on the medical center.

One off the Montefiore ASP's earliest multidisciplinary collaborations stemmed from an urgent need to improve Montefiore's performance on the community-acquired pneumonia (CAP) measure of the Centers for Medicare and Medicaid Services (CMS). In 2011, a quality improvement and stewardship intervention was implemented in collaboration with the ED involving a CAP bundle consisting of the following:

1. A CAP treatment algorithm for ED providers
2. A CAP kit with first-line antibiotics and dosing recommendations preloaded in the ED automated medication dispensing system
3. Audit of CAP antibiotics from an automated system

Although CMS compliance with antibiotic administration within 6 hours was no different before or after the intervention, a statistically significant improvement in appropriate CAP antibiotics was observed in the pilot ED because of the bundled intervention (improvement from 54.9% in 2008 to 93.4% in 2011, $P = .001$).[17]

In 2015 Montefiore established a multidisciplinary, transition-of-care outpatient parenteral antibiotic therapy (OPAT) program leveraging expertise in ID, stewardship, quality improvement, and patient safety. The program was designed to address safety concerns, high readmissions, and historically poor outcomes in patients discharged with IV catheters and extended IV antibiotics. The authors developed a treatment protocol adhering to the IDSA OPAT best practices and the OPAT care bundle published by Muldoon and colleagues[18] (appropriate patient selection, infectious diseases consultation, patient/caregiver education, discharge planning, outpatient monitoring/tracking, and a program outcomes review for optimization of patient care) and assessed its impact on hospital readmissions, ED utilization, and mortality over the course of a 6-month pilot period.

In addition to clinical monitoring, OPAT physicians serve as antimicrobial stewards by

1. Reviewing weekly laboratory results and drug levels
2. Contacting infusion teams and skilled nursing staff about therapeutic dose adjustments (eg, subtherapeutic vancomycin levels for methicillin-resistant *Staphylococcus aureus* infection requiring increase in dose)

3. Enacting IV to oral switch were appropriate
4. Determining ultimate duration of antibiotic therapy

Patients enrolled in the transition-of-care OPAT program had significantly fewer 30-day readmissions during the pilot period than those who received the previous standard of care (13.0% vs 26.1%, P<.01). The projected hospital savings from reduced readmissions was approximately $1 million in the first year of the program.[19]

Tracking and Reporting

Monitoring antibiotic prescribing patterns is essential for identifying targets for stewardship intervention, such as excessive use of costly agents and overly broad-spectrum antibiotics for a given indication. Furthermore, reporting patterns back to providers helps to reinforce best practices and identify and remedy any outliers.[8]

In 2010 to 2012 the Montefiore ASP partnered with 10 medical centers in the greater New York region to determine whether targeted stewardship interventions can result in a measurable reduction in hospital-onset C difficile infection (CDI) rates. Intervention facilities determined their top antibiotics linked to hospital-onset CDI using case control studies. Pre-intervention and postintervention hospital-onset CDI rates and antibiotic consumption were evaluated from June 2010 to January 2012. Defined daily dose, days of therapy (DOT), and number of antibiotic courses were also compared pre- and postintervention. Facilities identified piperacillin/tazobactam, fluoroquinolones, or cefepime as intervention targets given the high associated risk of CDI (odds ration 2.0–9.8). Facilities used several ASP interventions, particularly audit of prescriptions and feedback to prescribers. Total target antibiotic use significantly decreased when measured by DOT (P<.05). Intervention hospitals reported fewer hospital-onset CDI cases (2.8 rate point difference) compared with nonintervention hospitals; however, the project was unable to show statistically significant decreases in aggregate hospital-onset CDI either between intervention and nonintervention groups or within the intervention group over time. Although decreases in target antibiotic consumption did not translate into reductions of hospital-onset CDI, likely because of the multifactorial nature of CDI, there were several valuable lessons learned about ASP implementation and antibiotic use metrics. The findings helped establish ASP as a fundamental aspect of health care facility policy to control hospital-onset CDI. The study culminated in several publications and a national toolkit for reduction in CDI through stewardship.[20,21] It also served as a forerunner to future multicenter initiatives throughout NYC.

As members of the Healthcare Association of New York State (HANYS; a statewide hospital and continuing care association in New York promoting health care quality, education, and advocacy), the authors contributed Montefiore's 2015 antibiotic utilization data to the HANYS Antibiotic Stewardship Collaborative and received comparative data across multiple health care systems in NYS in the form of an antibiotic surveillance dashboard. The authors learned that between September and November 2015, Montefiore had an 8.09% antimicrobial utilization rate for piperacillin/tazobactam compared with a 6.16% rate among 39 reporting NYS hospitals. This finding catalyzed an intensive audit of piperacillin/tazobactam use to identify opportunities for de-escalation or cessation of therapy. From unit-level HANYS data, the authors were able to tailor interventions to specific front-line providers with particularly high piperacillin/tazobactam use. Participation in HANYS empowered the authors to provide valuable feedback on prescribing patterns to specific provider groups and present comprehensive data to the authors' administrators to help sustain and grow their stewardship program.

In 2018, Montefiore is participating in the Agency for Healthcare Research and Quality's Antibiotic Safety Program with the aim of augmenting auditing and reporting capabilities of participating hospital systems to meet important stewardship benchmarks of the CDC's National Healthcare Safety Network antibiotic use reporting program.

Education

Educational curriculum encompassing a range of inpatient and outpatient infections can positively impact prescribing behaviors when combined with other intensive stewardship interventions.[8] Active education with interactive tools, problem-based learning, and team-building exercises are gaining momentum across a range of learners, including medical students, residents, fellows, and mature clinicians.[7] Since inception of the Montefiore ASP in 2008, prescribers have benefited from tailored educational programs targeting learners at distinct levels. With assistance from multiple partners, novel programs were put into place highlighting the collaborative nature of the authors' ASP.

As part of a patient safety seminar for medical students at the Albert Einstein College of Medicine, the authors developed a case-based, interactive exercise introducing students to important concepts, such as infection prevention bundles, judicious prescribing, and transmission-based isolation precautions. The program was conceived to address knowledge gaps and introduce important patient safety principles at an earlier stage of professional training. Alongside their infection prevention colleagues, the authors demonstrated appropriate use of personal protective equipment (PPE), effective hand hygiene, and procedural safety techniques. Students practiced hand hygiene, PPE donning and doffing, and needle safety in breakout groups. A second complementary "Antibiotic Rally" seminar emphasized antibiotic resistance as a direct consequence of overprescribing in humans and livestock. In small groups, students were introduced to stewardship core activities and practiced use of antibiograms for bug-drug combinations. These sessions are highly regarded by both moderators and students and are among few medical school programs introducing stewardship and infection prevention in the preclinical curriculum.[7]

In collaboration with other stewardship and hospital epidemiology programs in NYC, the authors host an annual workshop in stewardship, infection prevention, and health care epidemiology sponsored by the Infectious Diseases Society of New York (IDSNY). The intended learners are senior ID fellows seeking to bolster stewardship and infection prevention acumen. Using a case-based format and interactive polling questions, the authors address challenging stewardship and infection prevention scenarios (emerging infections, drug shortages, occupational exposures, and so forth) and career development in stewardship, epidemiology, and public health. Participants engage in high-level discussions with a panel of experts from NYC hospital systems and the department of health.[7] The workshop is unique to the NYC region and is one of few similar programs across the country.

SUMMARY

On a daily basis, ASPs provide prescribing guidance, clinical decision support, education, and audit patterns of antimicrobial use throughout the hospital. ASPs also interface with health care facility leadership and external partners to support growth within the institution, garner regional and national recognition, and identify opportunities for scholarship, quality improvement, and research. Ideas for meaningful and impactful collaborations stem from daily interactions with colleagues, quarterly C-suite meetings, and national society meetings of like-minded individuals.

After an exploratory journey through innovative stewardship collaborations structured within the CDC's core elements framework, the authors present a final scenario highlighting a particularly rewarding and large-scale collaboration between NYC academic stewardship programs, microbiology colleagues, and the NYC Department of Health (NYCDOH).[22]

Antimicrobial stewardship vignette 2

In 2017, the authors' ASP and microbiology faculty partnered with the NYCDOH and neighboring stewardship programs in the Bronx, Manhattan, Queens, and Brooklyn to share regional antibiotic susceptibility data. The NYCDOH sought to develop a city-wide outpatient urinary tract antibiogram to assist community providers select appropriate antibiotic regimens for urinary tract infections and, therefore, assembled a consortium of experts in stewardship and clinical microbiology. Adult and pediatric susceptibility data on the 6 most prevalent outpatient urinary tract pathogens (*Enterobacter cloacae*, *Escherichia coli*, *Klebsiella pneumoniae*, *Proteus mirabilis*, *Pseudomonas aeruginosa*, and *Enterococcus faecalis*) were submitted from 16 medical centers. Data were compiled by the NYCDOH and presented electronically as borough-specific urinary tract antibiograms complete with an interpretation guide. ASP content experts contributed guidance on urinalysis interpretation and avoidance of asymptomatic bacteriuria. The end result was NYC's first regional antibiogram and comprehensive decision support tool to improve antibiotic appropriateness for urinary tract infections. The Montefiore ASP was proud to contribute and share their local susceptibility data for the benefit of prescribers and patients throughout NYC.

REFERENCES

1. Gratton L, Erickson TJ. Eight ways to build collaborative teams. Harvard Business Review 2007.
2. Ostrowsky B, Banerjee R, Bonomo RA, et al. Infectious diseases physicians: leading the way in antimicrobial stewardship. Clin Infect Dis 2018. https://doi.org/10.1093/cid/cix1093.
3. Rodriguez G, Yashayev R, Yushuvayev B, et al. A novel antimicrobial stewardship program-guided procalcitonin initiative for emergency department diagnosis of bacterial pneumonia in New York City. [abstract: 958]. IDWeek. San Diego, CA, October 3–7 2017.
4. Discussion and recommendations for the application of procalcitonin to the evaluation and management of suspected lower respiratory tract infections and sepsis. FDA executive summary. 2016. Available at: https://www.fda.gov/downloads/AdvisoryCommittees/CommitteesMeetingMaterials/MedicalDevices/MedicalDevicesAdvisoryCommittee/MicrobiologyDevicesPanel/UCM528156.pdf. Accessed May 31, 2018.
5. Schuetz P, Wirz R, Sager R, et al. Effect of procalcitonin-guided antibiotic treatment on mortality in acute respiratory infections: a patient level meta-analysis. Lancet Infect Dis 2018;18:95–107.
6. Pollack LA, Srinivasan A. Core elements of hospital antibiotic stewardship programs from the Centers for Disease Control and Prevention. Clin Infect Dis 2014;15(59):S97–100.
7. Nori P, Madaline T, Munjal I, et al. Developing interactive antimicrobial stewardship and infection prevention curricula for diverse learners: a tailored approach. Open Forum Infect Dis 2017;4(3):ofx117.

8. Barlam TF, Cosgrove SE, Abbo LM, et al. Implementing an antibiotic stewardship program: guidelines by the Infectious Diseases Society of America and the Society for Healthcare Epidemiology of America. Clin Infect Dis 2016;62(10):e51–77.

9. Nori P, Ostrowsky B, Dorokhova O, et al. Use of MALDI-ToF MS to resolve complex clinical cases of patients with recurrent bacteremias. J Clin Microbiol 2013; 51:1983–6.

10. Nori P, Szymczak W, Park C. Matrix-assisted laser desorption/ionization time-of-flight mass spectrometry (MALDI-ToF-MS) as a first line modality in the diagnosis of bacterial meningitis and septicemia – a report of five cases. Clin Microbiol Newsl 2016;38(7):57–60.

11. Morgan DJ, Malani P, Diekema DJ. Diagnostic stewardship—leveraging the laboratory to improve antimicrobial use. JAMA 2017;318(7):607–8.

12. Safyer SM. Montefiore-early and active on antimicrobial stewardship. Quality Collaborative. 2016. Available at: https://uhfnyc.org/assets/1473. Accessed February 20, 2018.

13. Trivedi KK, Ostrowsky B, Abbo LM, et al. Working together to define antibiotic appropriateness: point prevalence survey in 47 intensive care units from 12 US Hospitals, Partnership for Quality Care, March 2017. [abstract: 685]. IDWeek. San Diego, CA, 2017.

14. ASHP statement on the pharmacist's role in antimicrobial stewardship and infection prevention and control. Am J Health Syst Pharm 2010;67(7):575–7.

15. HIV/AIDS annual surveillance statistics. Available at: https://www1.nyc.gov/site/doh/data/data-sets/hiv-aids-annual-surveillance-statistics.page. Accessed February 20, 2018.

16. Guo Y, Chung P, Weiss C, et al. Customized order-entry sets can prevent antiretroviral prescribing errors: a novel opportunity for antimicrobial stewardship. P T 2015;40(5):353–60.

17. Ostrowsky B, Sharma S, DeFino M, et al. Antimicrobial stewardship and automated pharmacy technology improve antibiotic appropriateness for community-acquired pneumonia. Infect Control Hosp Epidemiol 2013;34(6): 566–72.

18. Muldoon EG, Snydman DR, Penland EC, et al. Are we ready for an outpatient parenteral antimicrobial therapy bundle? A critical appraisal of the evidence. Clin Infect Dis 2013;57(3):419–24.

19. Madaline T, Nori P, Mowrey W, et al. Bundle in the Bronx: impact of a transition-of-care outpatient parenteral antibiotic therapy bundle on all-cause 30-day hospital readmissions. Open Forum Infect Dis 2017;4(2). https://doi.org/10.1093/ofid/ofx097.

20. Ostrowsky B, Ruiz R, Brown S, et al. Preventing healthcare-associated infections: results and lessons learned from AHRQ's HAI program. Infect Control Hosp Epidemiol 2014;35(S3):S86–95.

21. AHRQ toolkit to reduce Clostridium difficile infections through stewardship. Available at: https://www.ahrq.gov/professionals/quality-patient-safety/patient-safety-resources/resources/cdifftoolkit/index.html. Accessed February 20, 2018.

22. 2016 New York City outpatient urinary tract antibiogram. Available at: nyc.gov/health/antibiogram. Accessed February 20, 2018.

Role of Education in Antimicrobial Stewardship

Inge C. Gyssens, MD, PhD[a,b,*]

KEYWORDS

- Responsible antibiotic use • Antimicrobial stewardship • Education • Postgraduate
- Undergraduate

KEY POINTS

- Education is the cornerstone of every antimicrobial stewardship program.
- Teaching of the principles of antimicrobial stewardship should start at the undergraduate level.
- Multidisciplinary input is needed for building the curricula in an attractive format.
- Strong political support is necessary for a curriculum program to be successfully implemented.

INTRODUCTION
Antimicrobial Resistance: An Unavoidable Threat

The ability to treat infectious diseases with antimicrobials is regarded as an essential component of medical management. The loss of antibiotics' effectiveness endangers routine medical and surgical procedures, including organ transplants and joint replacements. Timely administration of effective antibiotics; that is, antibiotics to which the causative pathogen is still susceptible, is crucial in the treatment of sepsis. In 2013, the Centers for Disease Control and Prevention (CDC) published a report outlining the top 18 drug-resistant threats to the United States. These threats were categorized based on level of concern: urgent, serious, and concerning.[1] In 2017, the World Health Organization published a list of the 12 pathogens that pose the greatest threat to human health because they are resistant to antibiotics (http://www.who.int/mediacentre/factsheets/fs194/en/). Novel antibiotics against these resistant organisms are needed. For many years, few new antibiotics with novel targets and mechanisms of action were in the research and development pipeline. Recently, there seems to be a

Disclosure Statement: There are no commercial of financial conflicts of interest for this article. No funding was obtained.

[a] Department of Medicine, Radboud University Medical Center, AIG 463, PO Box 9101, Nijmegen 6500 HB, The Netherlands; [b] Faculty of Medicine, Research Group of Immunology and Biochemistry, Hasselt University, Martelarenlaan 42, BE 3500, Hasselt, Belgium
* Department of Medicine, Radboud University Medical Center, AIG 463, PO Box 9101, Nijmegen 6500 HB, The Netherlands.
E-mail address: Inge.Gyssens@radboudumc.nl

Med Clin N Am 102 (2018) 855–871
https://doi.org/10.1016/j.mcna.2018.05.011
0025-7125/18/© 2018 Elsevier Inc. All rights reserved.

new interest by research and development companies to meet the need of antibiotics in the gram-negative spectrum.[2] Another problem is the recurring shortage of older, still-active antibiotics.[3]

The Common Good: Effective Antimicrobial Drugs

Antimicrobials differ from other drugs in a particular way. They are the only drugs that do not directly target the patient but instead inhibit or kill invading pathogens and commensal microorganisms. Antimicrobial therapy is not only based on the characteristics of a patient and a drug but also on the characteristics of the microorganisms and the colonizing flora causing the infection. A useful didactic tool that describes the complex interrelationship between humans, microorganisms, and antimicrobial drugs is the pyramid of infectious diseases (**Fig. 1**). Activity of the antimicrobial is obtained at the cost of the development of resistance by the pathogen, as well as in the microbiome. The selection of the appropriate antimicrobial therapy is a complex decision, depending on the knowledge of many different aspects of infectious diseases: immunologic and genetic host factors, microbial virulence, microbial resistance, and the pharmacokinetic-pharmacodynamic effects of drugs.

Due to the selection pressure on the environment, prescribers of antimicrobial drugs face an ethical dilemma when treating an individual patient with maximally broad empirical therapy to cover all potential pathogens. On the other hand, prescribers have a responsibility toward future generations to preserve the efficacy of antibiotics and minimize the development of resistance.[4] The former responsibility tends to promote overtreatment; the latter is usually overlooked. However, prudent antibiotic use is the only option to delay the emergence of resistance.

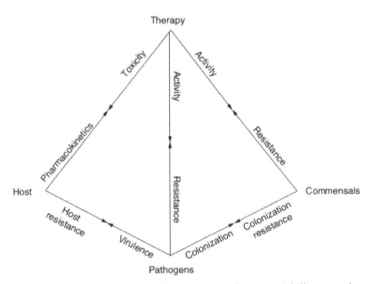

Fig. 1. Pyramid of infectious diseases. The arrows in the pyramid illustrate the multiple interactions between the patient, the drug, the pathogen or pathogens, and the colonizing microflora or microbiome. (*From* Pulcini C, Gyssens IC. How to educate prescribers in antimicrobial stewardship practices. Virulence 2013;4(2):193; with permission.)

Overuse and Underuse of Antimicrobial Drugs

Antibiotics are the most extensively developed and prescribed antimicrobial drugs. International comparative studies show that the quantity and quality of antibiotic prescribing differs greatly between countries. In Europe, there is a trend toward higher consumption in the north than in the south, and in the west than in the east.[5] For most countries, the prevalence of resistant pathogens follows the same pattern (https://ecdc.europa.eu/en/antimicrobial-resistance/surveillance-and-disease-data/data-ecdc). One of the major causes of overprescribing is insufficient knowledge of infectious diseases and the responsible use of antimicrobial drugs. More than 20 years ago, in 1993, the British Society of Antimicrobial Chemotherapy's Working Party on Antimicrobial Use considered training in infectious diseases and knowledge of prescribing of antimicrobial drugs was insufficient in clinicians.[6] In 2011, the Infectious Diseases Society of America (IDSA) stated:, clinician training and continuing education in appropriate antimicrobial use in the United States is "highly variable, non standardized, infrequent, and highly prone to bias, especially when conveyed or sponsored by pharmaceutical firms or their agents."[7] Conversely, focus on prescribing older, narrow-spectrum drugs in targeted therapy has been taught in medical schools and has been common practice in northern European countries where antimicrobial use is low, such as Scandinavia and the Netherlands, for several decades.[8] The role of up-to-date undergraduate and postgraduate education is even more important in low-income and middle-income countries, which are settings with restricted access to medical literature.[9]

In this article, relevant aspects of education for the health-care force are analyzed and discussed. The timeline and setting, the learning outcomes, and the format of education, as well as its evaluation, are explored. Education of the public is also considered important because patient participation in health care is receiving increasing attention. In the Western world, the highest volume of antibiotics is prescribed by health care practitioners, mostly physicians. It is, therefore, logical to focus primarily on the education of the prescribers of antibiotics.

EDUCATION ON ANTIMICROBIAL STEWARDSHIP PRINCIPLES BASED ON RESPONSIBLE ANTIMICROBIAL USE

According to IDSA, Antimicrobial stewardship includes not only limiting inappropriate use but also optimizing antimicrobial selection, dosing, route, and duration of therapy to maximize clinical cure or prevention of infection while limiting the unintended consequences, such as the emergence of resistance, adverse drug events, and cost.[10] AS is based on principles of responsible antibiotic use, a broad concept that was not clearly defined until recently. A recent review within the Driving Reinvestment in Research and Development (R&D) and Responsible Antibiotic Use (DRIVE-AB) project identified 17 synonyms of responsible antibiotic use. Following an extensive literature review and diverse stakeholder input, the DRIVE-AB consortium proposed a definition with 14 patient-level and 8 societal elements, as well as associated best-practice descriptions, for a global definition of responsible antibiotic use.[11] An important aspect of responsible antibiotic use is prudent antibiotic prescribing. **Table 1** presents the main principles for education in prudent antibiotic prescribing. The ultimate goal is to translate these principles into specific topics, concepts, disciplines, learning outcomes, and competencies for a core curriculum of medical doctors and other health care professionals. The program should cover the undergraduate level, the internship or foundation year, and specialty or professional training.

As an example, by applying the AS principles (see **Table 1**) in settings with a well-developed microbiology laboratory system, it is possible to adapt empirical therapy to a targeted therapy when culture results are known. This is called streamlining or deescalating antimicrobial therapy, and the strategy has become widely accepted because intensive care physicians[12] and even hematologists[13] have widely recommended it. Targeted therapy decreases unnecessary broad-spectrum antimicrobial exposure and results in cost containment. Deescalation may also include discontinuation of empirical antimicrobial therapy based on clinical criteria and negative culture results.[10]

Table 1
Principles of prudent antibiotic prescribing for education in Antimicrobial stewardship

Topic	Concept, Understanding	Field, Discipline	Principles, Learning Outcomes, Competencies
Bacterial resistance	Selection, mutation	Microbiology, genetics	• Extent, causes of bacterial resistance in pathogens (low antibiotic concentration, long-time exposure of microorganisms to antibiotics is driving resistance) • Extent, causes of bacterial resistance in commensals and the phenomenon of overgrowth (eg, *Clostridium difficile* infection, yeast infection)
		Epidemiology	• Epidemiology of resistance, accounting for local variations and importance of surveillance (differences between wards, countries)
	Hygiene	Infection control, mostly microbiology	• Spread of resistant organisms
Antibiotics	Mechanisms of action of antibiotics or resistance Toxicity	Pharmacology	• Broad-spectrum vs narrow-spectrum antibiotics, preferred choice of narrow-spectrum drugs • Combination therapy (synergy, limiting emergence of resistance, broaden the spectrum)
	Costs	Ethics, public health, pharmacology	• Collateral damage of antibiotic use (toxicity, cost) • Consequences of bacterial resistance • Lack of development of new antibiotics (limited arsenal)

(continued on next page)

Table 1 (continued)			
Topic	**Concept, Understanding**	**Field, Discipline**	**Principles, Learning Outcomes, Competencies**
Diagnosis of infection	Infection or inflammation	Physiology, microbiology, immunology, or infectious diseases	• Interpretation of clinical and laboratory biological markers • Fever and C-reactive protein elevation are also a sign of inflammation, not per se of an infection
	Isolation and identification of bacteria, viruses, and fungi	Microbiology	• Practical use of point-of-care tests (eg, urine dipstick, streptococcal rapid antigen diagnostic test in tonsillitis) • Importance of taking microbiological samples for culture before starting antibiotic therapy
	Susceptibility to antibiotics	Microbiology or infectious diseases	• Interpretation of basic microbiological investigations (Gram stain, culture, Polymerase chain reaction, serology)

Treatment of infection	Indication for antimicrobials	Clinical microbiology or infectious diseases
		Organ specialty
			• Definitions and indications of empiric or directed therapy vs prophylaxis
			• Clinical situations when not to prescribe an antibiotic
			  ○ Colonization vs infection (eg, asymptomatic bacteriuria)
			  ○ Viral infections (eg, acute bronchitis)
			  ○ Inflammation vs infection (eg, fever without a definite diagnosis in a patient with no severity criteria)

Prevention of infection	—	Pharmacotherapy, surgery, anesthesiology, clinical microbiology, or infectious diseases	• Surgical antibiotic prophylaxis: indication, choice, duration (short), timing
Medical record keeping	Choice Duration Timing	Clinical medicine	• Documentation of antimicrobial indication in clinical notes • Recording (planned) duration or stop date

(continued on next page)

Table 1
(*continued*)

Topic	Concept, Understanding	Field, Discipline	Principles, Learning Outcomes, Competencies
Prescribing antibiotics: initially	Empiric therapy (local guidelines, antibiotic booklets) Diagnostic uncertainty	Clinical microbiology, infectious diseases. or organ specialists Clinical pharmacology	• Best bacteriologic guess for empiric therapy • Choice in case of prior use of antibiotics when selecting an antibiotic for empiric therapy • Choosing the dose and interval of administration (basic principles of pharmacokinetic-pharmacodynamic effects) • Estimating the shortest possible adequate duration
Prescribing antibiotics: targeted therapy	Communication with the microbiology laboratory Value of specialist consultation in infectious diseases or microbiology	Clinical microbiology, infectious diseases, or organ specialists Hospital pharmacy	• Reassessment of the antibiotic prescription around day 3 • Streamlining or deescalation when microbiological results are known • Intravenous–oral switch (bioavailability of antibiotics) • Therapeutic drug monitoring to ensure adequate drug levels (eg, vancomycin)
Prescribing antibiotics: standard of care	The importance of guidelines in clinical practice Quality indicators of antibiotic use	Clinical medicine, organ specialists Quality institute	• Prescribing antibiotic therapy according to national or local practice guidelines • Audit and feedback assessing prescribing practice using quality indicators
Communication skills	Discussion techniques	Psychology, clinical medicine	• Explaining to the patient the absence of an antibiotic prescription • Education of patients regarding prudent antibiotic use (comply with the doctors' prescription, no self-medication)

From Pulcini C, Gyssens IC. How to educate prescribers in antimicrobial stewardship practices. Virulence 2013;4(2):195–6; with permission.

Education of the Professional in Antimicrobial Stewardship

In the medical community, antibiotics are prescribed universally by all doctors and dentists, unlike many other drugs for which prescribing is kept within a specialty (eg, neuroleptic drugs). In hospitals, most patients are treated for their infection by organ specialists. Only patients with complicated or severe infections will be referred to infectious diseases departments. In the European Center for Disease Prevention and Control's point prevalence survey on health care–associated infections and antimicrobial use report, the prevalence of patients receiving at least 1 antimicrobial agent was 35% (country range 21.4%–54.7%).[14] In the United States, the CDC reports that more than half of patients receive at least 1 antibiotic during their hospital stay.[15] Junior doctors of all specialties prescribe the antibiotics under the supervision of their seniors. Therefore, both senior and junior doctors must be educated so that this practice is changed.[16,17]

In some European countries (eg, the United Kingdom) clinical pharmacists, midwives, nurses, or physician assistants can also prescribe some antibiotics in selected clinical situations.[18] In the United States, nurse practitioners were found to have higher rates of antibiotic prescribing compared with physicians for pediatric patients with upper respiratory tract infections.[19] In addition, health professionals who do not prescribe also play a key role in AS. In the medical community, pharmacists dispense antimicrobials and advise patients. Therefore, all health care professionals who are in contact with the patient must be educated with respect to knowledge on antimicrobial resistance, evidence (or lack of evidence) of benefit of antibiotics in different conditions, knowledge of management of symptoms, and the use of microbiology laboratory tests to guide antibiotic treatment. Education on management of demanding patients is also required.[20] In hospitals, hospital pharmacists play a key role in the AS team in most AS programs.[10] An extensive review discussed the different components of AS in which microbiology laboratories and clinical microbiologists can make significant contributions to AS programs.[21] Recently, the unrecognized and underused role of the staff nurse in patient safety and organizational factors influencing antibiotic management were reviewed.[22,23] In long-term care facilities, tools integrated into the workflow of nurses were found to contribute to AS.[24] Thus, antibiotic management requires effective teamwork among all health professions. Finally, the antibiotic prescriptions for animals made by veterinarians and antibiotic use in agriculture practices must be considered. However, these topics are beyond the scope of this article.

Education is an essential element of any AS program. Educational interventions can be categorized as passive or active. Passive education alone (eg, lectures, educational events, leaflets, handouts), without active intervention, has been shown only marginally effective in changing antimicrobial prescribing practices and has no sustained impact.[10] Antibiotic guidelines are intended to improve the quality of care, to support public health decisions, to diminish unwanted diversity of practice, and to increase transparency (for the health care worker and the public). Guideline implementation can be facilitated through provider education and feedback on antimicrobial use and patient outcomes.[10] Clinical pathways have successfully been used to implement prudent antibiotic strategies, such as the deescalation pathway described by Singh and colleagues,[25] to curb inappropriate antibiotic use in the intensive care unit. Face-to-face and 1-to-1 educational sessions provided by physicians are based on established principles of behavioral science, market research, and communications theory. This type of education has been used intensively and successfully by the pharmaceutical industry. In a hospital-based study by Solomon and colleagues,[26] daily academic detailing reminded prescribing physicians to stop the use of previously started but unnecessary antibiotics. Participative physician feedback and multidisciplinary interventions have also been found to be effective methods to increase the judicious use of antibiotics and reduce costs.[27]

Considerable effort has been put into education trying to change the behavior of professionals. Up until now, most initiatives on education in AS have been deployed in the postgraduate setting in hospitals. Systematic reviews on interventions to change the prescribing behavior of professionals have been performed and updated by Davey and colleagues.[27–30] They critically appraised interventions using the 2015 Cochrane Effective Practice and Organisation of Care Group taxonomy. Educational components are identified in many types of interventions (**Table 2**). However, many intervention studies lack an appropriate study design and fail to show meaningful outcomes.[30] Some educational interventions are not successful.[31] The success may be limited owing to the rapid turnover of junior staff and the difficulty in maintaining a local continuous educational program.

Table 2
Educational components of interventions according to Effective Practice and Organisation of Care definitions

Intervention Function	Definition	Intervention Components
Education	Increasing knowledge or understanding	Educational meetings Dissemination of educational materials Educational outreach
Persuasion	Using communication to induce positive or negative feelings or to stimulate action	Educational outreach by academic detailing or review and recommend change
Restriction	Using rules to reduce the opportunity to engage in the target behavior (or increase the target behavior by reducing the opportunity to engage in competing behaviors)	Restrictive
Environmental restructuring	Changing the physical context	Physical reminders, such as posters, pocket-size or credit card-size summaries, or on laboratory test reports Structural (eg, new laboratory tests or rapid reporting of results)
Enablement	Increasing means or reducing barriers to increase capability or opportunity	Audit and feedback Decision support through computerized systems or through circumstantial reminders triggered by actions or events related to the targeted behavior Educational outreach by review and recommended change

From Davey P, Marwick CA, Scott CL, et al. Interventions to improve antibiotic prescribing practices for hospital inpatients. Cochrane Database Syst Rev 2017;2:CD003543; with permission.

Recently, the effect of education on the antibiotic management of special populations and specific topics has been studied using appropriate methodologies. Wei and colleagues[32] performed a cluster randomized trial on children with upper respiratory tract infections in primary care facilities in rural China. They obtained an intervention effect (absolute risk reduction in antibiotic prescribing) of -29% (95% CI -42 to -16, $P = 0.0002$). In France, the impact of implementing national prescribing guidelines for antibiotics in children was studied by an interrupted time series analysis. They showed significant decrease in the antibiotic prescription rate for acute respiratory tract infections and a dramatic drop in broad-spectrum antibiotic prescriptions.[33] Educational interventions have also targeted allergy history, resulting in improved allergy documentation.[34] In Spain, an educational AS program lowered the incidence and mortality rate of hospital-acquired candidemia and multiresistant drug bloodstream infection through sustained reduction in antibiotic use.[35]

Many national and international professional societies, organizations, and governmental bodies are deploying educational AS activities at the postgraduate level (**Box 1**).

Education of Medical and Other Trainees in Antimicrobial Stewardship

In the postgraduate training track, most medical and surgical specialties are anatomically defined but all prescribe antimicrobials. **Table 1** shows that the input of many disciplines is required to train a fellow at the bedside. The organ specialist (eg, urologist) may not have the fully required background for implementing the general principles of prudent antibiotic prescribing in the microbiological diagnostic and therapeutic

---

Box 1
Examples of educational activities in antimicrobial stewardship

The World Health Organization (WHO) chose antimicrobial resistance (AMR) as the topic for World Health Day in 2011 and put antimicrobial resistance on the health agenda of 129 WHO Member states. WHO has published its WHO competency framework for health workers' education and training on antimicrobial resistance in January 2018. Geneva: World Health Organization; 2018 (WHO/HIS/HWF/AMR/2018.1). Licence: CC BY-NC-SA 3.0 IGO.

In the United States, the IDSA published the white paper report "Bad Bugs, No Drugs" in 2004 and launched an advocacy campaign. In 2007, the IDSA and the Society for Healthcare Epidemiology of America (SHEA) issued guidelines for developing an institutional program to enhance antibiotic stewardship.[10] The American Society for Microbiology (ASM) has been organizing workshops in the topic of antimicrobial policies and stewardship before the Interscience Conference on Antimicrobial Agents and Chemotherapy (ICAAC) since 2004. Last year's ASM Microbe 2017 counted 5 different AS workshops.

The CDC started its campaign in 2010. Be Antibiotics Aware (formerly Get Smart about Antibiotics) is a national effort to help fight antibiotic resistance and improve antibiotic prescribing and use. It focuses on strategies to help inpatient health facilities implement interventions (https://www.cdc.gov/antibiotic-use/). The CDC collaborated with the SHEA to develop Core Elements of Hospital Antibiotic Stewardship Programs.[60]

In Europe, the European Centers for Disease Prevention and Control developed a toolkit consisting of evidence-based educational materials to support AS efforts at a national level [http://ecdc.europa.eu/en/EAAD/Pages/Home.aspx/]. The European Society on Clinical Microbiology and Infection (ESCMID) Study Group on Antimicrobial Stewardship (www.escmid.org/esgap) organized postgraduate international education courses before the ECCMID Conference.

management of urologic patients. In Canada, the CanMEDS Physician Competency framework describes the knowledge, skills, and abilities that specialist physicians need for better patient outcomes.[36] This model has been adapted around the world in the health profession. With worldwide increasing antibiotic resistance, national and local guidelines become paramount. Guidelines must be evidence-based, graded, and developed by a multidisciplinary group, involving all key stakeholders, to foster acceptance and ownership. National or international guidelines should be adapted to the local context to ensure relevance for local practice and policies. Transparency is key to promote confidence in the recommendations of the adapted guideline. Flexible, easily accessible formats must be used (eg, online tools, booklets, smartphone applications).

The format of internship or specialist training of medical doctors in Europe, the United States, and the world is variable regarding the onset of exposure to patients, the duration, the type of training, and the responsibilities. This renders standardization of learning outcomes difficult. The training period is extremely crucial for shaping behavior because junior doctors start to copy the behavior of their supervisors within the first weeks in the hospital.[16] Competencies and learning outcomes must be clearly defined. The impact of learning sessions can be enhanced by the measurement of current practice and the use of quality improvement strategies.[37,38] Recently, the training programs of graduated doctors into primary care or a specialty have been subject to reform in many countries. Silverberg and colleagues[39] reviewed the literature on AS training in 2016. They used Kirkpatrick's 4 levels of evaluation (ie, reaction, learning, behavior, and results) to categorize interventions. The investigators concluded that high-level evaluation was sparse, with 23% reporting a Kirkpatrick level 3 evaluation. Schrier and colleagues[40] described a format of AS educational curricula for pediatric trainees in Europe. A cross-sectional survey of pediatric residents at a US hospital assessed prescribing practices. Results showed the need for better use of clinical guidelines.[41] In Europe, Pulcini and colleagues[29] conducted a survey of doctors who were still in their training years in a French or a Scottish university hospital. Overall, 30% of those surveyed stated that they had had no training in antibiotic prescribing in the past year, although 99% had prescribed an antibiotic within the last 6 months. A reassuring feature was that 91% (France) and 97% (Scotland) cited guidelines as a factor that influenced their prescribing.[29]

In hospitals, a multidisciplinary AS team must be involved in the development and implementation of a local educational program for residents and fellows on prudent antibiotic prescribing. In the United States, the Joint Commission recently approved a new antimicrobial stewardship standard that contains statements on educating practitioners, staff, and patients on the AS program.[42]

Education of Undergraduate Students in Antimicrobial Stewardship

Many investigators have described the difficulties of changing the behavior of trained medical practitioners, with multiple barriers, including cultural.[43,44] Therefore, awareness has grown that starting the teaching of prudent antibiotic use at the undergraduate level might be more effective.[17]

Recently, the content, volume, and quality of undergraduate medical curricula teaching AS principles and resistance have been studied in a cross-sectional survey of 35 European medical schools in 13 European countries.[45] Prudent antibiotic use principles were taught in all but 1 medical school; however, only 4 of 13 countries had a national program. Interactive teaching formats were used less frequently than passive formats. The teaching was mandatory for 53% and started before clinical training in 71% of the courses. Wide variations in exposure of students to important principles of prudent antibiotic use were found among countries and within the same country. Some major principles were poorly covered (eg, reassessment and duration of antibiotic therapy, communication skills). Whereas 77% of the respondents (faculty) fully agreed that the teaching of these principles should be prioritized. However, lack of time, mainly due to rigid curriculum policies, was the main reported barrier to implementation. The investigators concluded that, given the study design, these are probably optimistic results.[45] In recent years, more information came available from surveys of medical schools in the United Kingdom and the United States. Castro-Sanchez and colleagues[46] performed a cross-sectional survey (80% response) of all undergraduate programs in human and veterinary medicine, dentistry, pharmacy, and nursing in the United Kingdom. Although most of the programs taught AS principles, only one-third included all recommended principles. Melber and colleagues[47] more specifically reviewed preclinical microbiology curricula among US medical schools. AS was addressed at 66% of institutions.

Indirect information on medical curricula is also available from a few surveys of medical students or junior doctors on perceptions, attitudes, and knowledge about antimicrobial prescribing practices.[29,48–50] In the United States, Minen and colleagues[48] surveyed medical students' perceptions and attitudes about their training on antimicrobial use to identify gaps in medical education in a university hospital. Abbo and colleagues[49] conducted a multicenter study at 2 US universities investigating fourth-year medical students' knowledge, attitudes, and perceptions about AS, as well as their perception of their preparedness to prescribe antimicrobials appropriately. Again, most of the students said that they would like more education on appropriate use of antimicrobials. Differences were found between medical schools in knowledge scores, educational resources used, perceived preparedness, and knowledge about antimicrobial use. One of the striking differences between the United States and European populations is that United States students did not mention local guidelines as resource for prescribing,[48] whereas British students are explicitly stimulated to prescribe according to local guidelines.[51] In Europe, in 2012, final-year students at 7 European medical schools participated in an online survey to learn about medical students' knowledge of and perspectives on antibiotic prescribing and resistance.[50] Again, most students wanted more education on choosing antibiotic treatments. Most thought that the antibiotics they would prescribe would contribute to resistance. Almost all (98%) thought that resistance would be a greater problem in the future.[50] In Australia, antimicrobial knowledge and confidence was surveyed in final-year medical students. Students were more likely to rate university education as sufficient for cardiovascular diseases (91%) compared with infectious diseases (72%). The investigators concluded that there was poor knowledge and confidence in infectious diseases, and recommended additional training in antimicrobial prescribing.[52]

The importance of undergraduate training in prudent prescribing of antibiotics has become increasingly recognized.[20] In the United Kingdom and Scotland, in particular, major efforts were made to adapt and revise undergraduate education on antibiotics. In the United Kingdom, the Specialist Advisory Committee on Antimicrobial Resistance (SACAR) has proposed to undertake the development of learning outcomes; that is, statements that indicate what a student should know, understand, and be able to do by the end of an educational program.[37] Prescribing is included as a component of the undergraduate program in the United Kingdom, and the importance of undergraduate training in prescribing is reflected in aspects of the General Medical Council (GMC) document, "Outcomes for Graduates (Tomorrow's Doctors)."[53] The GMC has endorsed the Royal Pharmaceutical Society's Competency Framework for all Prescribers.[51] This document contains two statement competencies relevant for antimicrobial prescribing ie, "Understands antimicrobial resistance and the roles of infection prevention, control and antimicrobial stewardship measures" and "Prescribes within relevant frameworks for medicines use as appropriate (eg, local formularies, care pathways, protocols and guidelines)."[51]

Reexamining the principles and learning outcomes in **Table 1**, it is clear that much emphasis is needed on the transfer of basic science knowledge at an early stage. The undergraduate curriculum and internship or foundation year seem optimal stages to build a solid knowledge base for later practice. For example, surgeons will have a much higher acceptance of prophylaxis guidelines if they have been exposed to the principles of guideline development and antibiotic prophylaxis when taught as core competencies in medical school. To reach this goal, strong input is needed from academia to transfer the knowledge in the undergraduate curriculum. As depicted in **Table 1**, a wide variety of disciplines must be involved, including epidemiology, ethics, and communication skills (eg, working with guidelines, communicating with the patient). To link the undergraduate and postgraduate programs, particularly in the period of internship or foundation training, close collaboration between health care providers and academicians, as well as between hospitals and medical schools, is needed.

In the undergraduate curriculum, classic formal lectures are seldom considered as a successful means of transferring knowledge. Over the past decade, problem-based learning has been introduced in many universities. This type of education allows for alternative formats of interactive learning in smaller student groups. It is important to identify the topics or concepts that benefit from a disease-oriented approach (eg, acute bronchitis) or problem-oriented approach (eg, antimicrobial resistance) rather than a pathogen-oriented approach (eg, methicillin-resistant Staphylococcus aureus [MRSA]) or a drug-oriented approach (eg, antibiotic classes). Microbial resistance can be part of microbiology teaching. Information on antibiotics can be part of pharmacology and managing the demands of patients (ie, parents of young children) can be integrated in communication skills sessions. However, targeted antibiotic sessions in the format of problem-based learning are absolutely necessary to integrate all aspects of the topic.[20] Apart from formal lectures, interactive learning with case vignettes, PowerPoint presentations, and role play can be particularly appropriate for this topic. Elective rather than core modules are particularly suitable for discussions in small groups. For example, suitable topics are case studies, with question-and-answer sessions, illustrating the evidence base of surgical prophylaxis. In a Canadian controlled pre-post study, a smartphone app was found to increase knowledge of prescribing of undergraduates in the context of local antimicrobial resistance patterns.[54] In the United States, an AS curriculum consisting of an online learning module and workshop significantly increased knowledge and attitudes toward collaborative AS among preclinical medical and pharmacy students.[55]

Strong political support is necessary for a curriculum program to be successfully implemented. As an example, in the United Kingdom, the GMC requested in 2009 that all postgraduate deans and Royal Colleges ensure that infection prevention, and control and antimicrobial prescribing, become standard practice implemented in all clinical settings, and ensure that they are strongly emphasized in undergraduate and postgraduate medical training.[38]

Education of the Public in Antimicrobial Stewardship

One could argue that in countries with a considerable over-the-counter antibiotic use, the patients share the responsibility of using antibiotics responsibly. However, even in the situation of over-the-counter purchases by the public, health professionals determine the purchasing behavior of the public because patients and providers tend to copy the doctor's prescribing choices.[56] In Europe, over-the counter-use by the public is low except for a few countries (eg, Romania, Greece, Cyprus, and Spain).[57,58] In the United States, a recent study on nonprescription antibiotics in primary care clinics showed that 5% of patients reported nonprescription use of systemic antibiotics in the last 12 months, 25% reported intended use, and 14% stored antibiotics at home. These rates were similar across race and ethnicity groups. The major source of antibiotics used without a prescription was a store or pharmacy in the United States (40%).[59]

SUMMARY

Education in AS is needed for the entire health-care force and the public. This education should start at an early stage in the undergraduate curriculum, to ensure maximal effect. In hospitals, the AS team must be involved in the development and implementation of a local educational program, not only for practicing clinicians but also for residents and fellows. Recently, efforts to obtain better insight into the knowledge gaps of trainees and undergraduate students, and forging the right attitudes at an early stage, are being deployed in many settings.

FUTURE CONSIDERATIONS

Multicenter studies should apply appropriate methods to demonstrate the effect of educational interventions, including meaningful outcomes. These methods include randomized controlled trials and quasiexperimental designs with time series analysis.

Curricula on AS are being revised worldwide; however, more robust evaluations of educational interventions and AS education of trainees are needed.

REFERENCES

1. Centers for Disease Control and Prevention. Antibiotic resistance threats in the United States, 2013. Available at: https://www.cdc.gov/drugresistance/threat-report-2013/pdf/ar-threats-2013-508.pdf. Accessed February 11, 2018.
2. Theuretzbacher U. Global antimicrobial resistance in gram-negative pathogens and clinical need. Curr Opin Microbiol 2017;39:106–12.
3. Pulcini C, Bush K, Craig WA, et al. Forgotten antibiotics: an inventory in Europe, the United States, Canada, and Australia. Clin Infect Dis 2012;54(2):268–74.
4. Leibovici L, Paul M, Ezra O. Ethical dilemmas in antibiotic treatment. J Antimicrob Chemother 2012;67(1):12–6.
5. Adriaenssens N, Coenen S, Versporten A, et al. European Surveillance of Antimicrobial Consumption (ESAC): outpatient antibiotic use in Europe (1997-2009). J Antimicrob Chemother 2011;66(Suppl 6): vi3–12.
6. Davey P, Hudson S, Ridgway G, et al. A survey of undergraduate and continuing medical education about antimicrobial chemotherapy in the United Kingdom. British Society of Antimicrobial Chemotherapy Working Party on Antimicrobial Use. Br J Clin Pharmacol 1993;36(6):511–9.
7. Spellberg B, Blaser M, Guidos RJ, et al. Combating antimicrobial resistance: policy recommendations to save lives. Clin Infect Dis 2011;52(Suppl 5):S397–428.

8. Halls GA. The management of infections and antibiotic therapy: a European survey. J Antimicrob Chemother 1993;31(6):985–1000.
9. Laxminarayan R, Duse A, Wattal C, et al. Antibiotic resistance-the need for global solutions. Lancet Infect Dis 2013;13(12):1057–98.
10. Dellit TH, Owens RC, McGowan JE Jr, et al. Infectious Diseases Society of America and the Society for Healthcare Epidemiology of America guidelines for developing an institutional program to enhance antimicrobial stewardship. Clin Infect Dis 2007;44(2):159–77.
11. Monnier AA, Eisenstein BI, Hulscher ME, et al. DRIVE-AB WP1 group. Towards a global definition of responsible antibiotic use: results of an international multidisciplinary consensus procedure. J Antimicrob Chemother 2018;73(suppl_6): vi3–16.
12. Borgatta B, Rello J. How to approach and treat VAP in ICU patients. BMC Infect Dis 2014;14:211.
13. Averbuch D, Orasch C, Cordonnier C, et al. European guidelines for empirical antibacterial therapy for febrile neutropenic patients in the era of growing resistance: summary of the 2011 4th European Conference on Infections in Leukemia. Haematologica 2013;98(12):1826–35.
14. European Center for Disease Prevention and Control. Point prevalence survey of healthcare-associated infections and antimicrobial use in European acute care hospitals 2011–2012. Available at: https://ecdc.europa.eu/sites/portal/files/media/en/publications/Publications/healthcae-associated-infections-antimicrobial-use-PPS.pdf. Accessed February 11, 2018.
15. Baggs J, Fridkin SK, Pollack LA, et al. Estimating national trends in inpatient antibiotic use among US hospitals from 2006 to 2012. JAMA Intern Med 2016; 176(11):1639–48.
16. De Souza V, MacFarlane A, Murphy AW, et al. A qualitative study of factors influencing antimicrobial prescribing by non-consultant hospital doctors. J Antimicrob Chemother 2006;58(4):840–3.
17. Pulcini C, Gyssens IC. How to educate prescribers in antimicrobial stewardship practices. Virulence 2013;4(2):192–202.
18. Dryden MS, Cooke J, Davey P. Antibiotic stewardship–more education and regulation not more availability? J Antimicrob Chemother 2009;64(5):885–8.
19. Ference EH, Min JY, Chandra RK, et al. Antibiotic prescribing by physicians versus nurse practitioners for pediatric upper respiratory infections. Ann Otol Rhinol Laryngol 2016;125(12):982–91.
20. Bond C. Education of patients and professionals. In: Gould IM, Van der Meer JWM, editors. Antibiotic policies. Theory and practice. New York: Kluwer Academic/Plenum Publishers; 2005.
21. Morency-Potvin P, Schwartz DN, Weinstein RA. Antimicrobial stewardship: how the microbiology laboratory can right the ship. Clin Microbiol Rev 2017;30(1): 381–407.
22. Monsees E, Goldman J, Popejoy L. Staff nurses as antimicrobial stewards: an integrative literature review. Am J Infect Control 2017;45(8):917–22.
23. Olans RN, Olans RD, DeMaria A Jr. The critical role of the staff nurse in antimicrobial stewardship–unrecognized, but already there. Clin Infect Dis 2016;62(1): 84–9.
24. Katz MJ, Gurses AP, Tamma PD, et al. Implementing antimicrobial stewardship in long-term care settings: an integrative review using a human factors approach. Clin Infect Dis 2017;65(11):1943–51.

25. Singh N, Rogers P, Atwood CW, et al. Short-course empiric antibiotic therapy for patients with pulmonary infiltrates in the intensive care unit. A proposed solution for indiscriminate antibiotic prescription. Am J Respir Crit Care Med 2000;162(2 Pt 1):505–11.

26. Solomon DH, Van Houten L, Glynn RJ, et al. Academic detailing to improve use of broad-spectrum antibiotics at an academic medical center. Arch Intern Med 2001;161(15):1897–902.

27. Davey P, Brown E, Fenelon L, et al. Interventions to improve antibiotic prescribing practices for hospital inpatients. Cochrane Database Syst Rev 2005;(4):CD003543.

28. Davey P, Brown E, Charani E, et al. Interventions to improve antibiotic prescribing practices for hospital inpatients. Cochrane Database Syst Rev 2013; 4:CD003543.

29. Pulcini C, Williams F, Molinari N, et al. Junior doctors' knowledge and perceptions of antibiotic resistance and prescribing: a survey in France and Scotland. Clin Microbiol Infect 2011;17(1):80–7.

30. Davey P, Marwick CA, Scott CL, et al. Interventions to improve antibiotic prescribing practices for hospital inpatients. Cochrane Database Syst Rev 2017;(2):CD003543.

31. Schwartz DN, McConeghy KW, Lyles RD, et al. Computer-assisted antimicrobial recommendations for optimal therapy: analysis of prescribing errors in an antimicrobial stewardship trial. Infect Control Hosp Epidemiol 2017;38(7): 857–9.

32. Wei X, Walley JD, Zhang Z, et al. Implementation of a comprehensive intervention for patients at high risk of cardiovascular disease in rural China: a pragmatic cluster randomized controlled trial. PLoS One 2017;12(8):e0183169.

33. Ouldali N, Bellettre X, Milcent K, et al. Impact of implementing national guidelines on antibiotic prescriptions for acute respiratory tract infections in pediatric emergency departments: an interrupted time series analysis. Clin Infect Dis 2017; 65(9):1469–76.

34. Krey SC, Waise J, Skrupky LP. Confronting the challenge of beta-lactam allergies: a quasi-experimental study assessing impact of pharmacy-led interventions. J Pharm Pract 2017. 897190017743154.

35. Molina J, Penalva G, Gil-Navarro MV, et al. Long-term impact of an educational antimicrobial stewardship program on hospital-acquired candidemia and multidrug-resistant bloodstream infections: a quasi-experimental study of interrupted time-series analysis. Clin Infect Dis 2017;65(12):1992–9.

36. Frank J, Snell L, Sherbino J, editors. CanMEDS 2015 physician competency framework. Ottawa (Canada): Royal College of Physicians and Surgeons of Canada; 2015. Available at: http://canmeds.royalcollege.ca/en/framework. Accessed February 11, 2018.

37. Davey P, Garner S. Professional education on antimicrobial prescribing: a report from the Specialist Advisory Committee on Antimicrobial Resistance (SACAR) professional education subgroup. J Antimicrob Chemother 2007;60(Suppl 1): i27–32.

38. McNulty CA, Cookson BD, Lewis MA. Education of healthcare professionals and the public. J Antimicrob Chemother 2012;67(Suppl 1):i11–8.

39. Silverberg SL, Zannella VE, Countryman D, et al. A review of antimicrobial stewardship training in medical education. Int J Med Educ 2017;8:353–74.

40. Schrier L, Hadjipanayis A, Del Torso S, et al. European Antibiotic Awareness Day 2017: training the next generation of health care professionals in antibiotic stewardship. Eur J Pediatr 2018;177(2):279–83.

41. Shukla PJ, Behnam-Terneus M, Cunill-De Sautu B, et al. Antibiotic use by pediatric residents: identifying opportunities and strategies for antimicrobial stewardship. Hosp Pediatr 2017;7(9):553–8.

42. The Joint Commission. New antimicrobial stewardship standard. 2017. Available at: https://www.jointcommission.org/assets/1/6/New_Antimicrobial_Stewardship_Standard.pdf. Accessed February 11, 2018.

43. Cabana MD, Rand CS, Powe NR, et al. Why don't physicians follow clinical practice guidelines? A framework for improvement. JAMA 1999;282(15):1458–65.

44. Hulscher ME, Grol RP, van der Meer JW. Antibiotic prescribing in hospitals: a social and behavioural scientific approach. Lancet Infect Dis 2010;10(3):167–75.

45. Pulcini C, Wencker F, Frimodt-Moller N, et al. European survey on principles of prudent antibiotic prescribing teaching in undergraduate students. Clin Microbiol Infect 2015;21(4):354–61.

46. Castro-Sanchez E, Drumright LN, Gharbi M, et al. Mapping antimicrobial stewardship in undergraduate medical, dental, pharmacy, nursing and veterinary education in the United Kingdom. PLoS One 2016;11(2):e0150056.

47. Melber DJ, Teherani A, Schwartz BS. A comprehensive survey of preclinical microbiology curricula among US medical schools. Clin Infect Dis 2016;63(2):164–8.

48. Minen MT, Duquaine D, Marx MA, et al. A survey of knowledge, attitudes, and beliefs of medical students concerning antimicrobial use and resistance. Microb Drug Resist 2010;16(4):285–9.

49. Abbo LM, Cosgrove SE, Pottinger PS, et al. Medical students' perceptions and knowledge about antimicrobial stewardship: how are we educating our future prescribers? Clin Infect Dis 2013;57(5):631–8.

50. Dyar OJ, Pulcini C, Howard P, et al. European medical students: a first multicentre study of knowledge, attitudes and perceptions of antibiotic prescribing and antibiotic resistance. J Antimicrob Chemother 2014;69(3):842–6.

51. Royal Pharmaceutical Society. A competency framework for all prescribers. 2016. Available at: https://www.rpharms.com/Portals/0/RPS%20document%20library/Open%20access/Professional%20standards/Prescribing%20competency%20framework/prescribing-competency-framework.pdf. Accessed February 11, 2018.

52. Weier N, Thursky K, Zaidi STR. Antimicrobial knowledge and confidence amongst final year medical students in Australia. PLoS One 2017;12(8):e0182460.

53. General Medical Council. Outcomes for graduates (Tomorrow's Doctors). 2015. Available at: https://www.gmcuk.org/education/undergraduate/undergrad_outcomes.asp. Accessed February 11, 2018.

54. Fralick M, Haj R, Hirpara D, et al. Can a smartphone app improve medical trainees' knowledge of antibiotics? Int J Med Educ 2017;8:416–20.

55. MacDougall C, Schwartz BS, Kim L, et al. An interprofessional curriculum on antimicrobial stewardship improves knowledge and attitudes toward appropriate antimicrobial use and collaboration. Open Forum Infect Dis 2017;4(1):ofw225.

56. Hadi U, Duerink DO, Lestari ES, et al. Survey of antibiotic use of individuals visiting public healthcare facilities in Indonesia. Int J Infect Dis 2008;12(6):622–9.

57. Grigoryan L, Monnet DL, Haaijer-Ruskamp FM, et al. Self-medication with antibiotics in Europe: a case for action. Curr Drug Saf 2010;5(4):329–32.

58. Guinovart MC, Figueras A, Llop JC, et al. Obtaining antibiotics without prescription in Spain in 2014: even easier now than 6 years ago. J Antimicrob Chemother 2015;70(4):1270–1.

59. Zoorob R, Grigoryan L, Nash S, et al. Nonprescription antimicrobial use in a primary care population in the United States. Antimicrob Agents Chemother 2016; 60(9):5527–32.

60. Centers for Disease Control and Prevention. Core elements of hospital antibiotic stewardship programs. Atlanta, 2016. Available at: https://www.cdc.gov/antibiotic-use/healthcare/pdfs/core-elements.pdf. Accessed February 11, 2018.

The Role of the Hospital Epidemiologist in Antibiotic Stewardship

Salma Abbas, MBBS[a], Michael P. Stevens, MD, MPH[b,c],*

KEYWORDS

- Antibiotic stewardship • Hospital epidemiology • Infection prevention
- Collaboration • Antibiotics

KEY POINTS

- Antibiotic stewardship programs (ASPs) are crucial to promote the judicious use of antibiotics.
- ASPs can prevent adverse events related to antibiotic use and lead to cost savings.
- There is great overlap between ASPs and infection control programs in terms of outcome measures, methodology, and technologies used. Integration of these programs can lead to synergy.
- Hospital epidemiologists can support ASPs by sharing data, collaborating on educational programs, helping to advocate for resources, and providing leadership.

INTRODUCTION

Multidrug-resistant organisms (MDROs), including methicillin-resistant *Staphylococcus aureus* (MRSA), vancomycin-resistant enterococci (VRE), and carbapenem-resistant Enterobacteriaceae pose a serious threat to health care today.[1,2] Although antibiotics have improved survival from life-threatening infections, injudicious use contributes to the emergence of MDROs.[1,3,4] Successful control and prevention of MDROs can be achieved through leadership commitment and investment in human

Disclosures: None.
Conflicts of Interest: None.
Funding Source: None.
[a] Division of Infectious Diseases, Virginia Commonwealth University, 1000 East Marshall Street, Suite 205, PO Box 980049, Richmond, VA 23298, USA; [b] Department of Hospital Epidemiology and Infection Control, Virginia Commonwealth University, North Hospital, 2nd Floor, Room 2-073, 1300 East Marshall Street, Richmond, VA 23298, USA; [c] Department of Infectious Diseases, Virginia Commonwealth University, North Hospital, 2nd Floor, Room 2-073, 1300 East Marshall Street, Richmond, VA 23298, USA
* Corresponding author. Virginia Commonwealth University, PO Box 980019, Richmond, VA 23298.
E-mail address: michael.stevens@vcuhealth.org

https://doi.org/10.1016/j.mcna.2018.05.002
0025-7125/18/© 2018 Elsevier Inc. All rights reserved.
medical.theclinics.com

and scientific resources.[2] Apart from MDROs, injudicious use of antimicrobials also contributes to *Clostridium difficile* infections (CDI).[5] According to a Centers for Disease Control and Prevention (CDC) estimate, approximately 30% to 50% of all antimicrobial use is either inappropriate or unnecessary.[3] The establishment of ASPs has been mandated for hospitals and nursing care centers in the United States by the Joint Commission.[6] Hospitals and health care systems should focus on developing infection control programs (ICPs) and ASPs led by physicians with specialized training in infectious diseases.[2] ICPs, led by hospital epidemiologists, are usually older and more established within hospitals. Given the overlap between ICP and ASP goals, metrics, and technologies, these programs present natural opportunities for synergy.

Evidence suggests that ASPs positively impact the quality of patient care and safety, decrease the likelihood of adverse events associated with antimicrobial use, improve infection cure rates, and decrease the rates of treatment failures through optimized use of antibiotics for treatment and prophylaxis.[3] Establishment of these programs has been shown to lower CDI rates, health care–associated infections (HAIs) caused by MDROs, and to reduce overall length of stay and associated costs.[3,7,8]

CORE ELEMENTS OF ANTIBIOTIC STEWARDSHIP PROGRAMS

Implementing ASPs is challenging, as prescribing practices and patient complexity vary across institutions.[3] There is no single format on which to base ASPs, and a one-size-fits-all strategy is not recommended, as institutional requirements differ.[3] Defined leadership and a multidisciplinary approach are recommended. Although ASPs likely will differ in terms of resources and activities, the CDC has outlined the following core elements for ASPs (**Table 1**)[3]:

- Leadership Commitment: Human, financial, and information technology resources should be allocated to ASPs.
- Accountability: A single leader should be appointed to lead ASPs. Evidence suggests that the presence of an infectious diseases physician is ideal.[1,9]

Table 1 Centers for Disease Control and Prevention core elements of antibiotic stewardship	
Leadership commitment	Allocate human, financial, and information technology resources to antibiotic stewardship programs (ASPs).
Accountability	A single leader should be appointed to lead ASPs. Ideally this would be an infectious diseases–trained physician.
Drug expertise	Appoint a single pharmacist leader to provide drug-related expertise.
Action	Active strategies, such as prior authorization, prospective audit, and feedback, and the use of antibiotic time-outs should be adapted.
Tracking	Antibiotic consumption and resistance patterns should be monitored. Antibiograms should be generated to reflect resistance profiles.
Reporting	Results of antimicrobial use and resistance profiles should be shared with relevant hospital staff members.
Education	Programs should be designed to educate prescribers regarding optimal antibiotic use.

Adapted from Centers for Disease Control and Prevention (CDC). Core elements of hospital antibiotic stewardship programs. Available at: https://www.cdc.gov/antibiotic-use/healthcare/implementation/core-elements.html. Accessed April 27, 2018.

- Drug Expertise: A single pharmacist leader should be appointed to provide drug expertise and help promote the judicious use of antibiotics.
- Action: Strategies such as evaluation of antimicrobial use at fixed intervals (also known as antibiotic time-outs), the use of antibiotic order forms, prior authorization, and prospective audit and feedback are recommended. These require review of antibiotics by an expert in antibiotic use to minimize unnecessary antibiotic prescriptions. Policies should be introduced in a stepwise fashion, beginning with passive measures, such as education, followed by active strategies, such as prospective audit and feedback.
- Tracking: Antibiotic consumption and resistance patterns should be monitored. Antibiograms should be generated to reflect resistance profiles.
- Reporting: Results of antimicrobial use and resistance profiles should be shared with physicians, nurses, and other relevant staff members.
- Education: Programs should be designed to educate prescribers regarding optimal antibiotic use.[1]

POLICIES TO OPTIMIZE ANTIBIOTIC USE

In addition to the core elements outlined in **Table 1**, ASPs should implement policies to minimize the unnecessary use of antimicrobial agents. These include the following[3]:

- Documentation of antibiotic dose, duration, and indication: this eliminates ambiguity and provides opportunities to correct the dose and duration for the intended indication.
- Developing institutional guidelines: these should follow national infection treatment guidelines for common infections but also reflect local resistance patterns and formulary options to guide clinical decision making.

COMPONENTS OF INFECTION CONTROL PROGRAMS

The World Health Organization (WHO) recommends that hospital administrators establish infection control committees that will inform the work of ICPs and allocate resources.[10] Infection control committees require representation from various disciplines including, but not limited to, nursing, pharmacy, microbiology, infectious diseases, housekeeping, engineering, and sterilization services.[10] A single member is appointed as the chairperson of the committee; this should be an individual who can directly access hospital administration. The recommended activities of ICPs include the following[10]:

- Implementing measures such as standard, contact, and other precautions as needed.
- Educating and training hospital staff members on optimal ICPs.
- Mandating measures, such as immunization, to promote the health of employees and protect against communicable diseases, such as viral hepatitis.
- Identifying hazards in the health care setting and minimizing risks to health care workers.
- Implementing measures, such as hand hygiene, aseptic techniques, single use of instruments, and the judicious use of antibiotics.
- Adopting policies to appropriately handle blood and body fluid exposures, used equipment, and medical waste.
- Using appropriate methods for environmental cleaning and collaborating with relevant support services, such as laundering facilities.
- Performing surveillance.

- Incident monitoring.
- Outbreak investigations.
- Reporting outcome and process data to hospital administrators.
- Conducting research.

The similarities between ICPs and ASPs are summarized in **Table 2**.

Table 2
Similarities between antibiotic stewardship programs and infection control programs

Similarities	Comments
Both require a multidisciplinary approach.	ICPs and ASPs include and collaborate with nursing, pharmacy, microbiology, information technology, and infectious diseases specialists, among others.
Both require accountability and leadership commitment.	Both ICPs and ASPs ideally report directly to senior hospital/health system leadership. Both ICPs and ASPs require direct financial support from the hospital/health system.
Both impact the quality of patient care and safety.	ICP activities extend to the patient care environment but also encompass, for example, the cleaning and disposal of equipment. ASP activities directly influence patient care.
Both use metrics tied to reimbursement. Both track outcome measures such as CDI rates and MDRO resistance patterns.	ICPs measure device-days, rates of HAIs, and LOS secondary to HAIs. ASPs track antibiotic use measures such as DOT per 1000 patient-days. ASPs also monitor resistance rates as well as CDI. Whereas ICPs typically only report on health care–associated infections, ASPs typically track resistance across all organisms.
Both are mandated in health care facilities.	ICPs have been subject to long-standing mandates, whereas ASP mandates were only deployed in the past few years.
Both require reporting outcomes. Audit and feedback are important techniques for both ICPs and ASPs.	ICPs base reporting on directly observed practices (such as compliance with hand hygiene), as well as documentation. ASPs use documentation to report outcomes.
Both can submit data to NHSN and receive benchmarked reports.	ICPs report HAI data directly to NHSN; data reporting is mandated for a number of HAIs. The AUR module allows ASPs to report antibiotic use data to NHSN and receive normalized, benchmarked antibiotic use reports. Reporting is not mandated for ASPs at this time.
Both are required to design educational programs for hospital staff.	As ICPs often have been in place longer and have long-standing educational programs, ICPs can assist ASPs in both the creation of educational programs and content and in their dissemination.
Both can conduct research/engage in quality improvement activities to promote program activities.	ICPs often have been in place longer, are better resourced, and have a history of deploying quality improvement projects. ASPs can benefit from ICP resources, experience, and leadership.

Abbreviations: ASP, antibiotic stewardship program; AUR, antibiotic use and resistance; CDI, *Clostridium difficile* infection; DOT, days of therapy; HAI, healthcare-associated infection; ICP, infection control program; LOS, length of stay; MDRO, multidrug-resistant organism; NHSN, National Healthcare Safety Network.

HOSPITAL EPIDEMIOLOGISTS AND ANTIBIOTIC STEWARDSHIP

The US health care system is subject to quality and reimbursement pressures.[7] The care delivery model has shifted from fee-for-service to reimbursement based on the quality of care.[7] Health care is tied to payment incentives for achieving or exceeding quality standards as well as penalties for falling short of established benchmarks.[7]

With the growing media interest in HAIs, external pressures, and the push for transparency, hospitals are now required by the Joint Commission and Centers for Medicare and Medicaid Services (CMS) to submit data on certain core metrics including catheter-associated urinary tract infections (CAUTIs), surgical site infections (SSIs), and central line–associated bloodstream infections, as well as infections caused by MDROs.[11] In 2008, CMS began withholding reimbursement for patients readmitted with certain HAIs.[11] This change in reimbursement, coupled with public reporting, heightened public awareness, and the increasing accountability of health care systems forced hospitals to expand ICPs focused on the prevention and monitoring of HAIs.[7,11] These models incentivize institutions to improve process and outcome measures in a cost-effective manner.[7] Moreover, the results of these may be used to support an institution's standing as a center providing quality care to patients.[7]

Currently, ICPs are affected by multiple external pressures, including legislative mandates, industry concerns, accrediting agencies, payers, professional societies, and consumer advocacy groups. These external pressures can sometimes be at odds with each other.[11] This is one of the biggest challenges faced by hospital epidemiologists today, and can lead to unnecessary antimicrobial use in an effort to prevent infections or comply with other external mandates. This may lead to the emergence of MDROs and higher rates of CDI, and contribute to costs, as well.[3,7,11] Quality and safety outcomes data for these elements are publicly reported.[7] ASPs, in collaboration with ICPs, help decrease antibiotic consumption, prevent the emergence of MDROs, and reduce CDI rates.[4,5] ASP metrics can target clinical outcomes and also can be used to directly support the mission of ICPs. This underscores the importance of collaboration between ASPs and ICPs.[1,4,9]

DEMONSTRATING THE VALUE OF STEWARDSHIP PROGRAMS TO HOSPITAL ADMINISTRATORS

The goal of ASPs is to improve clinical outcomes and to prevent the undesired effects of antibiotics such as toxicity and the emergence of MDROs. Designing and implementing ASPs to fit a given institution's needs and resources is challenging. Ideally, stewardship leaders should work directly with hospital administrators to determine goals, negotiate compensation, establish outcome measures, and identify resources required to successfully conduct stewardship activities.[1,7] Knowledge of outcome measures that institutions are evaluated against is critical so that ASPs may modify stewardship activities on an ongoing basis to meet institutional requirements.[7] Stewardship strategies can be implemented as components of infection control bundles.[7] Given the extensive net of ICPs in hospitals and the overlap of ICP and ASP goals, hospital epidemiologists can play a crucial role in furthering the mission of ASPs and demonstrating their value to hospital administrators. ASP initiatives should be shared with hospital staff, payers, and patients. They should be positioned such that they can contribute to improved clinical outcomes, such as lower CDI rates, as well as to decreased length of hospital stay. Additionally, ASP strategies can be linked to value-based purchasing and cost savings.[7]

REPORTING

The National Healthcare Safety Network (NHSN) was created by the CDC to track HAI data at the institution, state, region, and national levels. This allows ICPs to gauge the success of policies, compare results with other facilities, and identify areas for improvement.[12] The CDC introduced an antibiotic use and resistance (AUR) module as part of NHSN that collects and reports normalized antibiotic use data for a given institution with comparisons to other facilities.[3] At this time, reporting to the AUR module is not mandated. ICPs possess the knowledge and technical expertise to report to NHSN (as reporting of certain HAIs is mandated). Hospital epidemiologists and ICPs can assist ASPs by supporting their efforts with reporting to the AUR module. Additionally, hospital epidemiologists can share up-to-date institution-specific data regarding resistance patterns and HAI and CDI rates.[3] The infection control committee is an important venue where ASP reporting can occur. By reporting in this setting, ASPs can present data to key hospital stakeholders they otherwise may not be able to easily access. Hospital epidemiologists can facilitate ASP reporting at infection control meetings.

ANTIBIOGRAM DEVELOPMENT

ICPs work closely with microbiology departments and information technology services to generate local antibiograms. These are useful tools to recognize emerging resistance patterns among microorganisms and to guide empiric antimicrobial therapy (especially in the context of local treatment guidelines). Data should be organized in a tabular fashion with percentage susceptibilities reported separately for gram-positive and gram-negative organisms.[13] The data also may be categorized by patient locations, such as inpatient, outpatient, or at the hospital unit level.[13] Hospital epidemiologists can collaborate with the clinical microbiology laboratory to ensure timely generation and accessibility of antibiograms.[14] Once available, the results of antibiograms can be reflected in stewardship policies and local treatment algorithms and be shared with prescribers. This can be achieved through infection control committee meetings, nursing meetings, publishing on the hospital intranet, distribution of hard copies to relevant hospital employees, and so forth.[13] When published and disseminated in a timely fashion, antibiograms may improve hospital-wide empiric antibiotic prescription practices.[15]

SURVEILLANCE, DATA COLLECTION, AND PRESENTATION

Members of ICPs conduct surveillance, data collection, and analysis followed by presentation to a variety of audiences.[10] Hospital epidemiologists can assist ASPs by providing relevant data and also via sharing presentation templates and techniques.

Infection preventionists review clinical cultures as part of daily activities.[16] Surveillance methods include bedside rounding, manual chart reviews, and the use of electronic surveillance systems.[16] This presents an opportunity to communicate unusual resistance patterns and mismatches in antimicrobial susceptibility and prescribed antibiotics to ASP leaders and pharmacists. Hospital epidemiologists can play a role in bridging communication gaps between ASP members and ICPs.

EDUCATION AND TRAINING OF HOSPITAL STAFF MEMBERS

Infection control personnel are experienced and knowledgeable in their field. They are required to design educational programs for audiences from various backgrounds throughout the hospital. Hospital employees also may be sent to relevant off-site seminars or conferences.[17] WHO recommends developing an infection prevention manual that should be reviewed and periodically updated by the infection control committee.[10] This is an important educational tool that should be made accessible to hospital staff members. In addition to disseminating written guidelines, ICPs are also tasked with assessing the training needs of staff members and organizing awareness campaigns, training courses, and in-service educational programs on a regular basis.[10] Adherence to institutional practices is assessed on an ongoing basis and refresher courses should be provided as needed.[10] Hospital epidemiologists can incorporate elements of antibiotic stewardship into their infection control manuals as well as educational programs. This can familiarize hospital staff members with ASP policies and enhance ASP acceptance.[1] ASP educational materials should include updates on local prescription practices, resistance patterns, and recommended approaches to treating common infections, such as pneumonia, urinary tract infections (UTIs), skin and soft tissue infections (SSTIs), CDI, empiric treatment for MRSA infections, and the treatment of culture-proven infections.[3] Some examples of how ICPs can assist ASPs in designing and promoting educational materials are listed as follows:

- UTIs: Urine tests are often performed without appropriate indications and collection methods due to low costs and ready availability.[18] This results in antibiotic utilization driven by test results rather than symptoms and indications.[18] The overdiagnosis of UTIs impacts ICPs by falsely elevating CAUTI rates and leads to the inappropriate use of antibiotics, as well (thereby directly effecting ASPs). Hospital epidemiologists can create awareness and design educational programs for clinicians as well as nurses to ensure urine tests are ordered only when indicated and samples are collected as recommended.
- SSTIs: Patients with SSTIs often receive broad-spectrum antibiotics without a clear indication. A growing body of evidence suggests that broad-spectrum antibiotics can be avoided when treating these infections.[19,20] Stewardship interventions may result in an earlier switch from intravenous to oral antibiotics, less frequent use of antipseudomonal antibiotics, and fewer treatment complications.[19] SSTIs present an opportunity for hospital epidemiologists to help disseminate educational programs and materials to familiarize hospital staff members with the recommended antimicrobials for SSTIs. As ICPs already interface with hospital staff around health care–associated SSIs, optimal SSTI management is an important area in which ICPs and ASPs can synergize.
- MRSA therapy: Empiric anti-MRSA antibiotics are often initiated as indicated but continued despite negative cultures or the recovery of methicillin-susceptible *S aureus.* This practice can result in the suboptimal treatment of infection and poor outcomes.[21] Hospital epidemiologists can play a role in promoting the appropriate use of anti-MRSA antibiotics by sharing data with ASPs on local resistance patterns and also by developing protocols for MRSA surveillance and decolonization in the perioperative setting, where appropriate. ICPs can inform compliance with MRSA guidelines via educational programs for clinicians, pharmacists, and nursing staff.
- CDIs: Guidelines recommend discontinuation of all unnecessary antibiotics and proton pump inhibitors among patients with CDIs, but this does not always translate into practice.[3,5] CDI is associated with longer inpatient length of stay and health care costs.[3,5,22] CDI is an important outcome measure for both ICPs and ASPs and is an important area in which ICPs and ASPs can synergize, especially with the sharing of data and with educational programs.

- Surgical Prophylaxis: ASPs are tasked to develop guidelines for surgical prophylaxis to specify the choice and duration of antibiotics appropriate for the surgical site involved and recommend alternatives for special populations, including pediatric patients, immunosuppressed populations, and individuals with allergies.[23] Although perioperative antibiotics are often recommended for surgical prophylaxis, it is worth noting that they must be used in conjunction with measures such as preoperative bathing, skin preparation in the operating room, normothermia, and optimal glycemic control to optimally prevent SSIs. Perioperative antibiotics should be used only if indicated and should be administered in a fashion allowing optimal bactericidal concentrations in serum and tissue to be achieved at the time of surgery.[24] Hospital epidemiologists can conduct education and surveillance to ensure compliance with surgical prophylaxis guidelines and to avert adverse events associated with suboptimal antibiotic use.

SHARING OUTBREAK ALERTS WITH ANTIBIOTIC STEWARDSHIP PROGRAM TEAMS

Outbreaks may be caused by organisms commonly implicated in outbreaks such as MRSA and VRE, as well as unusual organisms including (but not limited to) multidrug-resistant tuberculosis, *Ewingella americana, Tsukamurella* species, *Rhodococcus bronchialis, Nocardia farcinica, Ewingella hormaechei, Acremonium kiliense, Malassezia pachydermatis, Curvularia lunata, Clostridium sordellii, Ochrobactrum anthropi*, and nontuberculous mycobacteria.[25] Management of outbreaks often requires modification of guidelines regarding infection control practices and antimicrobial therapy.[25] Hospital epidemiologists can share outbreak alerts with ASP teams to optimize outbreak control through monitoring and restriction of antibiotics in targeted units and implementing policies to prevent future outbreaks.[9]

ENGAGING FRONT-LINE NURSING STAFF IN ANTIBIOTIC STEWARDSHIP PROGRAMS

The role of nurses in ASPs has been recognized by the CDC. Nurses can contribute to stewardship in numerous ways: obtaining details of drug allergies on initial patient assessment, obtaining blood cultures before antibiotic administration, timely initiation of antibiotics in septic patients, adjustment and deescalation of antimicrobials by communicating microbiology results to physicians, monitoring for adverse events related to antibiotics, reviewing orders for antibiotics, performing "time-outs" and assessing the need for ongoing antibiotic use at predetermined time intervals, assessing for transition to oral antibiotics if applicable, patient education and medication reconciliation, and communication with staff at other facilities for change-over in the event that patients are transferred to a different hospital or long-term facility.[26] At present, nursing representation in stewardship programs is minimal and programs must be designed to increase awareness regarding antibiotic stewardship among nursing staff members.[26] Hospital epidemiologists collaborate with nursing leadership for most infection prevention campaigns. This partnership can serve as a bridge to engage nursing staff members with ASPs.

ASSISTANCE WITH INFORMATION TECHNOLOGY SUPPORT

ICPs use computer-based programs for surveillance, developing order sets, and modifying or restricting order entry. These programs may integrate input from various sources, such as microbiology, infection prevention, pharmacy, radiology, and clinical notes.[9,27] ASPs may benefit from these programs and use them for a variety of activities, including the review of antibiotic orders, with audit and feedback to providers, formulary authorization, antibiotic deescalation, and so forth.[27] The creation or adoption of these systems is an important area in which ASPs and ICPs can collaborate. Additionally, hospital epidemiologists and ICPs can support ASPs with the development of clinical decision algorithms, order sets, and order entry criteria for antibiotics within electronic medical record systems.

SUMMARY

Significant overlap exists between ASPs and ICPs. This overlap includes (but is not limited to) the use of various process and outcome metrics as well as information technology resources. Additionally, ASPs and ICPs both are subject to external pressures and mandates. As many ICPs are already firmly established within institutions, hospital epidemiologists can play an important role in familiarizing hospital staff members with the goals of ASPs and can help ASPs gain local buy-in and support. This may be achieved through activities such as the development of local guidelines; training and education of staff; rounding with medical teams to assess compliance with ASP and infection prevention policies; bridging gaps between ASPs and departments, such as nursing, microbiology, and information technology; sharing surveillance data; providing assistance with presenting and reporting data; and the development of local antibiograms. Collaboration between ASPs and ICPs likely will lead to synergy with resultant optimized patient outcomes and safety.

REFERENCES

1. Dellit TH, Owens RC, McGowan JE, et al. Society for Healthcare Epdemiology of America Guidelines for Developing an Institutional Program to Enhance Antimicrobial Stewardship. Clin Infect Dis 2007;44(2):159–77.
2. Centers for Disease Control and Prevention. Available at: https://www.cdc.gov/infectioncontrol/pdf/guidelines/mdro-guidelines.pdf. Accessed May 29, 2018.
3. Centers for Disease Control and Prevention. Available at: Centers for Disease Control and Prevention. Available at: https://www.cdc.gov/antibiotic-use/healthcare/implementation/core-elements.html. Accessed May 29, 2018.
4. Moody J, Cosgrove SE, Olmstead R, et al. Antmicrobial stewardship: a collaborative partnership between infection preventionists and healthcare epidemiologists. Infect Control Hosp Epidemiol 2012;33(4):328–30.
5. Centers for Disease Control and Prevention. Available at: https://www.cdc.gov/hai/organisms/cdiff/cdiff_infect.html. Accessed May 29, 2018.
6. Approved New Antimicrobial Stewardship Standard. The Joint Commission. Available at: https://www.jointcommission.org/assets/1/6/New_Antimicrobial_Stewardship_Standard.pdf. Joint Commission Perspectives 2016;36(7):1–4. Accessed May 29, 2018.
7. Nagel JL, Stevenson JG, Eiland EH, et al. Demonstrating the value of antimicrobial stewardship programs to hospital administrators. Clin Infect Dis 2014;59(3):146–53.
8. Karnika S, Paudel S, Grigoras C, et al. Systematic review and meta-analysis of clinical and economic outcomes from the implementation of hospital-based antimicrobial stewardship programs. Antimicrob Agents Chemother 2016;60(8):4840–52.
9. MacDougall C, Polk RE. Antimicrobial stewardship programs in health care systems. Clin Microbiol Rev 2005;18(4):636–56.
10. The World Health Organization. Available at: http://www.wpro.who.int/publications/docs/practical_guidelines_infection_control.pdf. Accessed May 29, 2018.

11. Snydor EMR, Perl TM. Hospital epidemiology and infection control in acute-care settings. Clin Microbiol Rev 2011;24(1):141–73.
12. Centers for Disease Control and Prevention. Available at: https://www.cdc.gov/nhsn/about-nhsn/index.html. Accessed May 29, 2018.
13. Joshi S. Hospital antibiogram: a necessity. Indian J Med Microbiol 2010;28(4):277–80.
14. Diekema DJ, Saubolle MA. Clinical microbiology and infection prevention. J Clin Microbiol 2011;49(9):S57–60.
15. Furuno JP, Comer AC, Johnson JK, et al. Using antibiograms to improve antibiotic prescribing in skilled nursing facilities. Infect Control Hosp Epidemiol 2014;35(3):56–61.
16. Hsu HE, Shenoy ES, Kelbaugh D, et al. An electronic surveillance tool for catheter-associated urinary tract infection in intensive care units. Am J Infect Control 2015;43(6):592–9.
17. Morikane K. Infection control in healthcare settings in Japan. J Epidemiol 2012;22(2):86–90.
18. Pallin DJ, Ronan C, Montazeri K, et al. Urinalysis in acute care of adults: pitfalls in testing and interpreting results. Open Forum Infect Dis 2014;1(1):ofu019.
19. Gibbons JA, Smith HL, Kumar SC, et al. Antimicrobial stewardship in the treatment of skin and soft tissue infections. Am J Infect Control 2017;45(11):1203–7.
20. Pallin DJ, Camargo CA Jr, Schuur JD. Skin infections and antibiotic stewardship: analysis of emergency department prescribing practices, 2007-2010. West J Emerg Med 2014;15(3):282–9.
21. The Infectious Diseases Society of America. Available at: http://www.idsociety.org/uploadedFiles/IDSA/Manage_Your_Practice/Archived_Content/Quality_Improvement/QI_Measures_Concepts/Appropriate%20Use%20of%20Anti-MRSA%20Antibiotics%20JUNE2016.pdf. Accessed May 29, 2018.
22. Miller AC, Polgreen LA, Cavanaugh JE, et al. Hospital *Clostridium difficile* infection rates and prediction of length of stay in patients without *C. difficile* infection. Infect Control Hosp Epidemiol 2016;37(4):404–10.
23. Bratzler DW, Dellinger EP, Olsen KM, et al. Clinical practice guidelines for antimicrobial prophylaxis in surgery. Am J Health Syst Pharm 2013;70(3):195–283.
24. Berríos-Torres SI, Umscheid CA, Bratzler DW. Centers for Disease Control and Prevention Guideline for the prevention of surgical site infection, 2017. JAMA Surg 2017;152(8):784–91.
25. Archibald LK, Jarvis WR. Health care-associated infection outbreak investigations by the Centers for Disease Control and Prevention, 1946-2005. Am J Epidemiol 2011;174(11 Suppl):47–64.
26. American Nursing Association. Available at: http://www.nursingworld.org/ANA-CDC-AntibioticStewardship-WhitePaper. Accessed May 29, 2018.
27. Morency-Potvin P, Schwartz DN, Weinstein RA. Antimicrobial stewardship: how the microbiology laboratory can right the ship. Clin Microbiol Rev 2017;30(1):381–407.

Role of the Clinical Microbiology Laboratory in Antimicrobial Stewardship

Emilio Bouza, MD, PhD[a,b,c,d],*, Patricia Muñoz, MD, PhD[a,b,c,d],
Almudena Burillo, MD, PhD[a,b,c]

KEYWORDS

- Antimicrobial stewardship • Microbiology • Rapid diagnosis
- Clinical laboratory techniques • Laboratory organization

KEY POINTS

- The microbiology department should be able to systematically select patients who will benefit from microbiological information and assigned proactively to a fast track protocol.
- The microbiology department should develop diagnostic routines for same-day reporting and implement rapid identification and antimicrobial susceptibility testing procedures for special patients and samples.
- The microbiology red phone is made up of a medical microbiologist and all the information the laboratory must make sure is reported to clinicians during the critical period of management.
- The microbiology department should put into practice the rapid reporting of results and create an alliance with clinical pharmacy and the antimicrobial stewardship committee to influence the adequate prescription of antibiotics.

INTRODUCTION

The support offered by a microbiology department to an antimicrobial stewardship program depends on the department's infrastructure and functioning. Among the factors that affect the contribution to the program of this department, are its capacity to offer its services 24 hours a day/7 days a week, the training of its members, and their

Disclosure statement: The authors have no conflict of interest to declare.
a Medicine Department, School of Medicine, Universidad Complutense de Madrid (UCM), Plaza Ramón y Cajal s/n, Madrid 28040, Spain; b Instituto de Investigación Sanitaria Gregorio Marañón, Doctor Esquerdo, 46, Madrid 28007, Spain; c Department of Clinical Microbiology and Infectious Diseases, Hospital General Universitario Gregorio Marañón, Doctor Esquerdo 46, Madrid 28007, Spain; d CIBER de Enfermedades Respiratorias (CIBERES CB06/06/0058), Doctor Esquerdo 46, Madrid 28007, Spain
* Corresponding author. Department of Clinical Microbiology and Infectious Diseases, Hospital General Universitario Gregorio Marañón, Doctor Esquerdo 46, Madrid 28007, Spain.
E-mail address: emilio.bouza@gmail.com

Med Clin N Am 102 (2018) 883–898
https://doi.org/10.1016/j.mcna.2018.05.003
0025-7125/18/© 2018 Elsevier Inc. All rights reserved.

medical.theclinics.com

knowledge of clinical issues. The success of any such program also depends on the receptiveness of responsible physicians to the information and advice offered by the microbiology staff throughout the day. There is, therefore, no universal formula applicable to all these departments. From the perspective of our general hospital with a 24-hour microbiology laboratory service, we describe the clinical competencies of our antimicrobial stewardship program, including what we believe is a feasible model at present. These contributions are reported as 10 action points that can be used as a guideline.

SYSTEMATIC SELECTION OF PATIENTS WHO WILL ESPECIALLY BENEFIT FROM MICROBIOLOGICAL INFORMATION AND WILL BE PROACTIVELY ASSIGNED BY THE MICROBIOLOGIST TO A FAST TRACK PROTOCOL

All clinical samples submitted to the laboratory cannot be given the same priority or diagnostic preference. This means that the laboratory itself needs to have the capacity to identify patients who will benefit from rapid proactive action. In our department, we have discussed what the best warning criteria might be for selecting patients who are likely to benefit from a fast track approach. Some of these criteria are listed in **Box 1**.

These patients should be assigned to a microbiologist guide, or better, to a multidisciplinary work group that will be in charge of managing all their samples, provide rapid diagnoses, and suggest possible procedures. This person or workgroup will inform the responsible physician of any diagnostic developments within the first 8 hours, both positive and negative. The workgroup described herein is called the microbiology red phone in our institution.

RAPID REPORTING OF POSITIVE AND NEGATIVE TEST RESULTS: MICROBIOLOGY RED PHONE

Communication with clinicians is essential[1] and a particular section of the laboratory should be responsible for providing such preferential information. We call this section the microbiology red phone. The section is made up of a medical microbiologist who coordinates all requests for rapid information from clinicians and all the information the laboratory must make sure is reported to clinicians during the critical period of management. Ideally, the section is functionally equipped with a pharmacy service representative and an infectious diseases physician.[2] Its work is carried out by telephone and it can also promote the consultations conducted at the bedside, alerting infectious

---

Box 1
Selection criteria for patients requiring a "fast track" microbiology laboratory approach

Patients should meet at least 1 of the following criteria:

1. Be hospitalized or pending hospitalization, have blood cultures requested and in process (negative until now), and have other samples sent that same day to the laboratory for diagnosis (eg, urine, respiratory samples, cerebrospinal fluid, usually sterile fluids, tissue samples, etc) on which it is possible to work with rapid techniques.

2. Be admitted to an intensive care unit.

3. Be admitted to a unit for transplanted, immunocompromised, or hematooncology patients.

4. Be assigned to a fast track approach at the discretion of the responsible physicians or the infectious diseases department.

5. Patients with sepsis alert.

diseases consultants. This information group also spares the rest of the microbiology laboratory from typical interruptions during routine work and serves as a bridge between each clinician and each laboratory bench. Some activities of our red phone section are listed in **Box 2**.

SPEEDING UP THE LABORATORY WORKUP OF SAMPLES OF PARTICULAR SIGNIFICANCE

Clinical samples on which a rapid diagnosis must be made are variable, and so are the ways to speed up the diagnosis. Here are just a few examples of how diagnostic routines within a context of antimicrobial stewardship can be expedited. A recent advance is the possibility of confirming or excluding a diagnosis of influenza virus or respiratory syncytial virus (RSV) in less than 1 hour.[3–5] In our opinion, these results can influence antimicrobial stewardship by adding a laboratory message. In the event that results for influenza virus and RSV are both negative, the results offered may be followed by the message, "Consider suspending oseltamivir or other antiinfluenza agent if started." A positive flu result could prompt the message, "Consider suspending antibacterial treatment if initiated in this patient." Further, in patients in whom RSV is detected and the flu test result is negative, the message from the laboratory could be, "Consider suspending both antiinfluenza treatment such as oseltamivir and antibacterial treatment." This new flu test based on nucleic acid detection at a reasonable laboratory price has been a significant advance in recent years.[6–11]

We now describe an example of how routine urocultures can be improved and streamlined in hospitalized patients. Hospitalized patients for whom a urine culture has been requested and blood cultures have been also requested in the same working day are selected from the laboratory's work list. This is a list of patients with suspected urinary sepsis. Our routine work consists of immediately subjecting these urine samples to a Gram stain and then conducting direct identification using matrix-assisted laser desorption/ionization time of flight (MALDI-TOF) analysis on urine samples with visible microorganisms. We also add the molecular detection of carbapenemases for patients with microorganisms potentially carrying these enzymes. In all these patients, a preliminary direct antibiogram on the urine sample is started, which will provide highly reliable data over the following 18 hours.[12] At the end of this process and within 4 hours of submitting the urine and blood samples, the clinician receives telephone information about the findings accompanied by empirical therapeutic advice.

Box 2
Some responsibilities of the microbiology red phone

1. Direct reporting to doctors of patients with positive blood cultures.

2. Sepsis alert to all doctors and nurses of patients from whom blood cultures have been obtained.

3. Warn of rapid results (negative or positive) for usually sterile samples and discuss the implications of these results with the clinicians in charge.

4. Calls to the caregivers of patients with multidrug-resistant microorganisms and triggering of the immediate isolation procedures.

5. Direct oral reporting (besides electronic reporting) of positive results of particular relevance to ensure the information reaches the responsible clinician. An example would be a phone call to inform of the isolation of *Mycobacterium tuberculosis* complex both to the physicians and the epidemiology and prevention chain.

In the following sections, we detail what the microbiology laboratory can do to rapidly search for specific pathogens and possible impacts on the use of antimicrobials.

RAPIDLY SEARCHING FOR CERTAIN PATHOGENS

Rather than providing an exhaustive description of all potential laboratory tests that could have an impact on antimicrobial stewardship, we only give a few examples targeting each group of microorganisms. We have already mentioned the great usefulness in the field of virology of an immediate influenza and RSV test during the seasonal incidence of these agents. Another example is the cerebrospinal fluid screening test for herpes simplex virus, which is often performed in patients with suspected meningitis or cerebrospinal fluid encephalitis. We and other groups have argued a very low profitability of this test in patients with cellularly and biochemically normal cerebrospinal fluid. The information by telephone that the performance of the test is not appropriate, or that the result is negative, translates to considerable savings in the unnecessary use of acyclovir.[13–15]

For the detection of a *Staphylococcus aureus* carrier state, if we consider tests designed to quickly detect bacteria, a paradigmatic example is the use of rapid tests, which can be carried out directly on clinical samples in less than 2 hours. Several authors have shown that a negative test result reasonably allows for the exclusion of this microorganism as a causal agent of pneumonia in the patient and this finding should have immediate impacts in avoiding or suspending antistaphylococcal antimicrobial agents, and particularly agents against methicillin-resistant *S aureus*.[16–25] The detection of Gram-negative carbapenemase-producing bacilli in direct clinical samples, carriers, or patients, as well as in laboratory isolates, has a very clear impact on the clinical management of these patients and on avoiding the unnecessary use of toxic and expensive drugs.[26–29]

A molecular test for the *Clostridium difficile* toxin gene, when negative, means that *C difficile* can be reasonably ruled out as a causative agent in a patient with symptoms of diarrhea, and this will also guide the search for other agents, thus avoiding the unnecessary use of expensive antibiotics such as fidaxomicin. In contrast, in patients testing positive for the gene, the threshold cycle of the toxin gene amplification curve is a surrogate marker of toxin quantity and can help to identify patients at high risk of recurrence who would be candidates for fidaxomicin as a first-choice agent.[30–33]

In the field of tuberculosis, today's molecular techniques allow for the confirmation in hours of the presence of *Mycobacterium tuberculosis*, but also inform of the possibility of resistance to rifampicin that is frequently associated with resistance to isoniazid.[34–39]

In a setting of antifungal stewardship, the role of the microbiology laboratory can be equally relevant. The rapid use of biomarkers of fungal infection such as *Candida albicans* germ tube antibody, mannan antigens, antimannan antibodies, and $(1\rightarrow3)$-β-d-glucan, *Candida* spp. polymerase chain reaction, or T2 MRI for *Candida* diagnosis, allow us to work on patients who have received empirical antifungals for suspected invasive candidiasis.[40–48] The negativity in the first 5 days of all these tests enables a recommendation to suspend any antifungals with a high degree of safety. In the future, we should be able to custom design the duration of invasive candidiasis treatment for patients with this infection.

RAPID ANTIMICROBIAL SUSCEPTIBILITY TESTING

We have discussed the usefulness of antibiotic tests carried out directly on the clinical specimen received, without waiting for bacterial isolation and the standard performance of these tests. In our laboratory, these rapid tests are used routinely in patients with suspected pneumonia associated with mechanical ventilation. When added to the use of chromogenic agars, these tests are extraordinarily practical for providing a reliable antibiogram within 18 hours of incubation. The rapid reporting to intensivists of this information has a clear impact on the unnecessary use of antibiotics.[49,50]

The rapid antibiogram with a long-standing tradition of using E-test strips and impregnated discs directly on the broths of positive blood cultures, and a whole set of new technology including new microfluid techniques will rapidly become common laboratory practice, able to report susceptibility in less than 5 hours.[51–64] We also recommend rapid antibiograms directly on urine samples in hospitalized patients with suspected urinary sepsis. We should nevertheless insist that this area of work must be coordinated by a special group in charge of these patients with the essential feature of direct verbal communication with the clinician.[65–70]

The rapid antimicrobial sensitivity tests that are already being used combining microscopy and MALDI-TOF identification are set to offer susceptibility data within 8 hours of receiving a sample, in the near future.[71–77]

It is important to remember that it is not necessary to treat all positive cultures, particularly if they represent colonization with saprophytic flora, or contamination from a nonsterile source.[78]

SYSTEMATIC SEARCH FOR CONFLICTIVE PATHOGENS

Microorganisms that need to be routinely searched for in different samples and patient groups have not yet been precisely defined and each hospital and service has its own preferences. As an example, we comment on some of the circumstances that we believe may have the greatest impact on antimicrobial policy.

The detection of carrier status of *S aureus* has been discussed elsewhere in this article. Nasal sample detection is considered sufficiently representative of body colonization status, although the inclusion of surveillance in other regions undoubtedly increases its efficiency. Culture-based tests can lead to a delay of 48 hours in the availability of information and, in our opinion, it is preferable to use molecular tests so that information may be available in less than 2 hours.[20,22,25,79–81] The nasal decontamination of carriers has proven effective at reducing infections in patients undergoing cardiac surgery, although its impact is not so evident in patients scheduled for a prosthetic joint implantation.[82–85] In patients testing positive, decontamination should be initiated ideally within 5 days of the surgical procedure, but patients are often admitted shortly before surgery, thus preventing the implementation of this precaution. We recommend systematic performing of the nasal *S aureus* test in these 2 patient populations with direct information given to the clinician.

Rectal swab screening for multidrug-resistant Gram-negative bacilli is recommended for patients from other health care facilities with a history of carrying multidrug-resistant bacteria or who have recently received antimicrobials.[86–93]

We do not recommend the systematic search for *C difficile* toxin in patients without diarrhea, but some Canadian hospitals have reported favorable results of this type of screening and detecting carriers from their time of admission to hospital. These patients will be particularly susceptible to episodes of *C difficile*-associated diarrhea in case of use of antimicrobials for any indication.[94–97]

Recent data question the systematic search for *Candida* spp. carrier status in patients in the intensive care unit, given the lack of evidence that early therapy in colonized patients is associated with a decrease in mortality.[98] We have confirmed the usefulness of systematically searching for influenza virus in patients admitted to critical care units during the flu season, because it has served to identify many unsuspected cases of flu, even in patients with well-documented bacterial infections. In these circumstances, lower respiratory tract samples are as or more useful than classic nasopharyngeal samples.[4,99]

RAPID DETECTION OF RESISTANCE

We have discussed the possibility of quickly determining the sensitivity or resistance of different bacteria or fungi to antimicrobial agents, both using tests based on micro-cultures and microscopy and tests carried out directly on clinical samples. As particularly promising, we would like to highlight the possibility of immediate sensitivity results through mass spectrometry and other techniques (MALDI-TOF-MS).[100–114] As far as we are aware, no major studies have examined the impacts of the immediate availability of results in clinical practice. What we do know is that this impact depends not only on the given test's performance, but also on the ability to communicate its results to a clinical board via the person who has the knowledge to do so. This is an activity that we also entrust to our red phone section.

ALLIANCE WITH CLINICAL PHARMACY AND THE STEWARDSHIP COMMITTEE TO INFLUENCE PRESCRIPTION: CHECKLISTS

As mentioned elsewhere in this article, it is essential to carry out programs based on hospital pharmacy and microbiology department databases to detect errors in clinical practice and implement alerts.[115] In the context of antibacterial stewardship, combining information on antibiotic prescription versus isolation sensitivity in microbiology is a continuous source of intervention programs.[115–127]

Many programs are based on alerting physicians who prescribe broad-spectrum or restricted antimicrobials without requiring diagnostic microbiological testing. This type of program can work automatically and practically without verbal intervention. Programs that warn of antibiotic treatments that are not active against the isolated pathogen are more specific. An example of this is the dissociation between beta-lactam use in patients with bacteremia owing to methicillin-resistant S aureus, or glycopeptides in patients with bacteremia owing to methicillin-susceptible S aureus.[128] This type of situation requires not only an online warning, but also a telephone call and confirmation of receipt of the alert. A program of particular interest is the decrease in the unnecessary use of carbapenemics in patients not colonized with isolations of multidrug-resistant microorganisms.

We have discussed the suspension of antifungals in patients with negative biomarkers after 5 days of treatment and recommendations associated with the influenza/RSV test during the seasonal periods of these diseases.

STATISTICS FOR CLINICIANS AND EPIDEMIOLOGISTS: THE STEWARDSHIP COMMITTEE

One of the obligations of microbiology is to keep statistical information based on its databases to guide stewardship programs. Tables of the microorganisms most frequently isolated in the different samples and their antimicrobial sensitivity should be provided at intervals of no longer than 6 months and subdivided particularly for some units, such as critical care, according to their particular data.[129]

Microbiology can also provide trend indices of different processes based exclusively on their data, which should be calculated not only in general terms, but also specifically for different groups. In **Box 3**, we provide an example of some variables derived from microbiological data that can be offered by the laboratory.

Box 3
Examples of microbiological indices of trends in hospital infections

1. Trend by 1000 admissions of episodes of nosocomial bacteremia.

2. Trend of nosocomial bacteremia by multidrug-resistant Gram-positive and Gram-negative organisms per 1000 admissions.

3. Trend in catheter-related bacteremia per 1000 admissions. Includes patients with blood cultures and catheter tips positive for the same microorganism.

4. Trend shown by methicillin-resistant *Staphylococcus aureus* per 1000 microbiological sample isolates.

5. Trend shown by isolates of BGN multidrug-resistant organisms per 1000 microbiological samples.

6. Episodes of invasive candidiasis per 1000 admissions.

7. Episodes of candidemia per 1000 DDD of echinocandins.

8. Episodes of bacteremia owing to methicillin-resistant *S aureus* per 1000 DDD of glycopeptides + oxadolidinones.

9. Episodes of multidrug-resistant gram-negative bacteremia per 1000 DDD of carbapenemics.

10. Number of interventions per 1000 entries from the microbiology hotline.

PERIODIC MEETINGS WITH GROUPS OF PHYSICIANS AND NURSES

Microbiology must leave the laboratory and become physically visible to the doctors and nurses of the institution. That is why we believe that the department should, at least once a year, visit the units, both in the hospital and beyond that submit more samples to the laboratory. This visit should consist of sharing available microbiology data on available tests from microbiology in relation to the visited department, exploring opportunities for improvement, and discussing problems that the unit has in relation to the microbiology department. This feedback should then be used to establish ways of collaboration to address specific problems. The visit can be shared with other members of the antimicrobial stewardship team, particularly specialists in infectious diseases, pharmacy, infection prevention and control specialists, and hospital epidemiologists. The participation of the microbiology department in antimicrobial stewardship is an excellent way to establish its role as a key service that is much more than a diagnostic laboratory and has implications for patient morbidity and mortality as well as institution spending.

ACKNOWLEDGMENTS

The authors thank Ana Burton for her help in the preparation of the article.

REFERENCES

1. Simoes AS, Couto I, Toscano C, et al. Prevention and control of antimicrobial resistant healthcare-associated infections: the microbiology laboratory rocks! Front Microbiol 2016;7:855.

2. MacVane SH, Hurst JM, Steed LL. The role of antimicrobial stewardship in the clinical microbiology laboratory: stepping up to the plate. Open Forum Infect Dis 2016;3(4):ofw201.

3. Lopez Roa P, Catalan P, Giannella M, et al. Comparison of real-time RT-PCR, shell vial culture, and conventional cell culture for the detection of the pandemic influenza A (H1N1) in hospitalized patients. Diagn Microbiol Infect Dis 2011; 69(4):428–31.

4. Lopez Roa P, Rodriguez-Sanchez B, Catalan P, et al. Diagnosis of influenza in intensive care units: lower respiratory tract samples are better than nose-throat swabs. Am J Respir Crit Care Med 2012;186(9):929–30.

5. Gonzalez-Del Vecchio M, Catalan P, de Egea V, et al. An algorithm to diagnose influenza infection: evaluating the clinical importance and impact on hospital costs of screening with rapid antigen detection tests. Eur J Clin Microbiol Infect Dis 2015;34(6):1081–5.

6. Dugas AF, Valsamakis A, Gaydos CA, et al. Evaluation of the Xpert Flu rapid PCR assay in high-risk emergency department patients. J Clin Microbiol 2014;52(12):4353–5.

7. Haglund S, Quttineh M, Nilsson Bowers A, et al. Xpert Flu as a rapid diagnostic test for respiratory tract viral infection: evaluation and implementation as a 24/7 service. Infect Dis (Lond) 2018;50(2):140–4.

8. Soto M, Sampietro-Colom L, Vilella A, et al. Economic impact of a new rapid PCR assay for detecting influenza virus in an emergency department and hospitalized patients. PloS One 2016;11(1):e0146620.

9. Sendi P, Egli A, Dangel M, et al. Respiratory syncytial virus infection control challenges with a novel polymerase chain reaction assay in a tertiary medical center. Infect Control Hosp Epidemiol 2017;38(11):1291–7.

10. Cohen DM, Kline J, May LS, et al. Accurate PCR detection of influenza A/B and respiratory syncytial viruses by use of cepheid Xpert Flu+RSV Xpress assay in point-of-care settings: comparison to prodesse ProFlu. J Clin Microbiol 2018; 56(2) [pii:e01237-17].

11. Antoniol S, Fidouh N, Ghazali A, et al. Diagnostic performances of the Xpert((R)) Flu PCR test and the OSOM((R)) immunochromatographic rapid test for influenza A and B virus among adult patients in the Emergency Department. J Clin Virol 2018;99-100:5–9.

12. Burillo A, Rodriguez-Sanchez B, Ramiro A, et al. Gram-stain plus MALDI-TOF MS (matrix-assisted laser desorption ionization-time of flight mass spectrometry) for a rapid diagnosis of urinary tract infection. PloS One 2014;9(1):e86915.

13. Lopez Roa P, Alonso R, de Egea V, et al. PCR for detection of herpes simplex virus in cerebrospinal fluid: alternative acceptance criteria for diagnostic workup. J Clin Microbiol 2013;51(9):2880–3.

14. Hauser RG, Campbell SM, Brandt CA, et al. Cost-effectiveness study of criteria for screening cerebrospinal fluid to determine the need for herpes simplex virus PCR testing. J Clin Microbiol 2017;55(5):1566–75.

15. Van TT, Mongkolrattanothai K, Arevalo M, et al. Impact of a rapid herpes simplex virus PCR assay on duration of acyclovir therapy. J Clin Microbiol 2017;55(5): 1557–65.

16. Rocha LA, Marques Ribas R, da Costa Darini AL, et al. Relationship between nasal colonization and ventilator-associated pneumonia and the role of the environment in transmission of Staphylococcus aureus in intensive care units. Am J Infect Control 2013;41(12):1236–40.

17. Dangerfield B, Chung A, Webb B, et al. Predictive value of methicillin-resistant Staphylococcus aureus (MRSA) nasal swab PCR assay for MRSA pneumonia. Antimicrob Agents Chemother 2014;58(2):859–64.

18. Langsjoen J, Brady C, Obenauf E, et al. Nasal screening is useful in excluding methicillin-resistant Staphylococcus aureus in ventilator-associated pneumonia. Am J Infect Control 2014;42(9):1014–5.
19. Rimawi RH, Ramsey KM, Shah KB, et al. Correlation between methicillin-resistant Staphylococcus aureus nasal sampling and S. aureus pneumonia in the medical intensive care unit. Infect Control Hosp Epidemiol 2014;35(5): 590–3.
20. Johnson JA, Wright ME, Sheperd LA, et al. Nasal methicillin-resistant Staphylococcus aureus polymerase chain reaction: a potential use in guiding antibiotic therapy for pneumonia. Perm J 2015;19(1):34–6.
21. Giancola SE, Nguyen AT, Le B, et al. Clinical utility of a nasal swab methicillin-resistant Staphylococcus aureus polymerase chain reaction test in intensive and intermediate care unit patients with pneumonia. Diagn Microbiol Infect Dis 2016;86(3):307–10.
22. Baby N, Faust AC, Smith T, et al. Nasal methicillin-resistant Staphylococcus aureus (MRSA) PCR testing reduces the duration of MRSA-targeted therapy in patients with suspected MRSA pneumonia. Antimicrob Agents Chemother 2017;61(4) [pii:e02432-16].
23. Smith EA, Gold HS, Mahoney MV, et al. Nasal methicillin-resistant Staphylococcus aureus screening in patients with pneumonia: a powerful antimicrobial stewardship tool. Am J Infect Control 2017;45(11):1295–6.
24. Smith MN, Erdman MJ, Ferreira JA, et al. Clinical utility of methicillin-resistant Staphylococcus aureus nasal polymerase chain reaction assay in critically ill patients with nosocomial pneumonia. J Crit Care 2017;38:168–71.
25. Parente DM, Cunha CB, Mylonakis E, et al. The clinical utility of methicillin resistant Staphylococcus aureus (MRSA) nasal screening to rule out MRSA pneumonia: a diagnostic meta-analysis with antimicrobial stewardship implications. Clin Infect Dis 2018. https://doi.org/10.1093/cid/ciy024.
26. Peter H, Berggrav K, Thomas P, et al. Direct detection and genotyping of Klebsiella pneumoniae carbapenemases from urine by use of a new DNA microarray test. J Clin Microbiol 2012;50(12):3990–8.
27. Burillo A, Marin M, Cercenado E, et al. Evaluation of the Xpert Carba-R (Cepheid) assay using contrived bronchial specimens from patients with suspicion of ventilator-associated pneumonia for the detection of prevalent carbapenemases. PloS One 2016;11(12):e0168473.
28. Walker CD, Shankaran S. Extended antibiotic resistance in carbapenemase-producing Klebsiella pneumoniae: a case series. Am J Infect Control 2016; 44(9):1050–2.
29. Su CF, Chuang C, Lin YT, et al. Treatment outcome of non-carbapenemase-producing carbapenem-resistant Klebsiella pneumoniae infections: a multicenter study in Taiwan. Eur J Clin Microbiol Infect Dis 2017. https://doi.org/10.1007/s10096-017-3156-8.
30. Reigadas E, Alcala L, Valerio M, et al. Toxin B PCR cycle threshold as a predictor of poor outcome of Clostridium difficile infection: a derivation and validation cohort study. J Antimicrob Chemother 2016;71(5):1380–5.
31. Senchyna F, Gaur RL, Gombar S, et al. Clostridium difficile PCR cycle threshold predicts free toxin. J Clin Microbiol 2017;55(9):2651–60.
32. Kamboj M, Brite J, McMillen T, et al. Potential of real-time PCR threshold cycle (CT) to predict presence of free toxin and clinically relevant C. difficile infection (CDI) in patients with cancer. J Infect 2017. https://doi.org/10.1016/j.jinf.2017.12.001.

33. Dionne LL, Raymond F, Corbeil J, et al. Correlation between Clostridium difficile bacterial load, commercial real-time PCR cycle thresholds, and results of diagnostic tests based on enzyme immunoassay and cell culture cytotoxicity assay. J Clin Microbiol 2013;51(11):3624–30.

34. Watanabe Pinhata JM, Cergole-Novella MC, Moreira dos Santos Carmo A, et al. Rapid detection of Mycobacterium tuberculosis complex by real-time PCR in sputum samples and its use in the routine diagnosis in a reference laboratory. J Med Microbiol 2015;64(9):1040–5.

35. Mutingwende I, Vermeulen U, Steyn F, et al. Development and evaluation of a rapid multiplex-PCR based system for Mycobacterium tuberculosis diagnosis using sputum samples. J Microbiol Methods 2015;116:37–43.

36. Scherer LC, Sperhacke RD, Rossetti ML, et al. Usefulness of the polymerase chain reaction dot-blot assay, used with Ziehl-Neelsen staining, for the rapid and convenient diagnosis of pulmonary tuberculosis in human immunodeficiency virus-seropositive and -seronegative individuals. Infect Dis Rep 2011; 3(1):e3.

37. Perez-Garcia F, Ruiz-Serrano MJ, Lopez Roa P, et al. Diagnostic performance of Anyplex II MTB/MDR/XDR for detection of resistance to first and second line drugs in Mycobacterium tuberculosis. J Microbiol Methods 2017;139:74–8.

38. Bunsow E, Ruiz-Serrano MJ, Lopez Roa P, et al. Evaluation of GeneXpert MTB/RIF for the detection of Mycobacterium tuberculosis and resistance to rifampin in clinical specimens. J Infect 2014;68(4):338–43.

39. Alonso M, Navarro Y, Barletta F, et al. A novel method for the rapid and prospective identification of Beijing Mycobacterium tuberculosis strains by high-resolution melting analysis. Clin Microbiol Infect 2011;17(3):349–57.

40. Escribano P, Marcos-Zambrano LJ, Gomez A, et al. The Etest performed directly on blood culture bottles is a reliable tool for detection of Fluconazole-resistant Candida albicans isolates. Antimicrob Agents Chemother 2017;61(7) [pii: e00400-17].

41. Martinez-Jimenez MC, Munoz P, Valerio M, et al. Combination of Candida biomarkers in patients receiving empirical antifungal therapy in a Spanish tertiary hospital: a potential role in reducing the duration of treatment. J Antimicrob Chemother 2016;71(9):2679.

42. Leon C, Ruiz-Santana S, Saavedra P, et al. Contribution of Candida biomarkers and DNA detection for the diagnosis of invasive candidiasis in ICU patients with severe abdominal conditions. Crit Care 2016;20(1):149.

43. Martinez-Jimenez MC, Munoz P, Valerio M, et al. Combination of Candida biomarkers in patients receiving empirical antifungal therapy in a Spanish tertiary hospital: a potential role in reducing the duration of treatment. J Antimicrob Chemother 2015;70(11):3107–15.

44. Martinez-Jimenez MC, Munoz P, Valerio M, et al. Candida biomarkers in patients with candidaemia and bacteraemia. J Antimicrob Chemother 2015;70(8): 2354–61.

45. Martin-Mazuelos E, Loza A, Castro C, et al. beta-D-Glucan and Candida albicans germ tube antibody in ICU patients with invasive candidiasis. Intensive Care Med 2015;41(8):1424–32.

46. Mylonakis E, Zacharioudakis IM, Clancy CJ, et al. The efficacy of T2 magnetic resonance assay in monitoring Candidemia after the initiation of antifungal therapy: the serial therapeutic and antifungal monitoring protocol (STAMP) trial. J Clin Microbiol 2018. https://doi.org/10.1128/JCM.01756-17.

47. Zervou FN, Zacharioudakis IM, Kurpewski J, et al. T2 magnetic resonance for fungal diagnosis. Methods Mol Biol 2017;1508:305–19.

48. Mylonakis E, Clancy CJ, Ostrosky-Zeichner L, et al. T2 magnetic resonance assay for the rapid diagnosis of candidemia in whole blood: a clinical trial. Clin Infect Dis 2015;60(6):892–9.

49. Cercenado E, Cercenado S, Marin M, et al. Evaluation of direct E-test on lower respiratory tract samples: a rapid and accurate procedure for antimicrobial susceptibility testing. Diagn Microbiol Infect Dis 2007;58(2):211–6.

50. Bouza E, Torres MV, Radice C, et al. Direct E-test (AB Biodisk) of respiratory samples improves antimicrobial use in ventilator-associated pneumonia. Clin Infect Dis 2007;44(3):382–7.

51. Malmberg C, Yuen P, Spaak J, et al. A novel microfluidic assay for rapid phenotypic antibiotic susceptibility testing of bacteria detected in clinical blood cultures. PloS One 2016;11(12):e0167356.

52. Rodel J, Bohnert JA, Stoll S, et al. Evaluation of loop-mediated isothermal amplification for the rapid identification of bacteria and resistance determinants in positive blood cultures. Eur J Clin Microbiol Infect Dis 2017;36(6):1033–40.

53. Arroyo MA, Denys GA. Parallel evaluation of the MALDI sepsityper and verigene BC-GN assays for rapid identification of gram-negative Bacilli from positive blood cultures. J Clin Microbiol 2017;55(9):2708–18.

54. Verroken A, Defourny L, le Polain de Waroux O, et al. Clinical impact of MALDI-TOF MS identification and rapid susceptibility testing on adequate antimicrobial treatment in sepsis with positive blood cultures. PloS One 2016;11(5):e0156299.

55. Rodel J, Karrasch M, Edel B, et al. Antibiotic treatment algorithm development based on a microarray nucleic acid assay for rapid bacterial identification and resistance determination from positive blood cultures. Diagn Microbiol Infect Dis 2016;84(3):252–7.

56. Jayol A, Dubois V, Poirel L, et al. Rapid detection of polymyxin-resistant enterobacteriaceae from blood cultures. J Clin Microbiol 2016;54(9):2273–7.

57. Foschi C, Compri M, Smirnova V, et al. Ease-of-use protocol for the rapid detection of third-generation cephalosporin resistance in Enterobacteriaceae isolated from blood cultures using matrix-assisted laser desorption ionization-time-of-flight mass spectrometry. J Hosp Infect 2016;93(2):206–10.

58. Barnini S, Brucculeri V, Morici P, et al. A new rapid method for direct antimicrobial susceptibility testing of bacteria from positive blood cultures. BMC Microbiol 2016;16(1):185.

59. Sothoron C, Ferreira J, Guzman N, et al. A Stewardship approach to optimize antimicrobial therapy through use of a rapid microarray assay on blood cultures positive for gram-negative bacteria. J Clin Microbiol 2015;53(11):3627–9.

60. Nagel JL, Huang AM, Kunapuli A, et al. Impact of antimicrobial stewardship intervention on coagulase-negative Staphylococcus blood cultures in conjunction with rapid diagnostic testing. J Clin Microbiol 2014;52(8):2849–54.

61. Hill JT, Tran KD, Barton KL, et al. Evaluation of the nanosphere Verigene BC-GN assay for direct identification of gram-negative bacilli and antibiotic resistance markers from positive blood cultures and potential impact for more-rapid antibiotic interventions. J Clin Microbiol 2014;52(10):3805–7.

62. Sango A, McCarter YS, Johnson D, et al. Stewardship approach for optimizing antimicrobial therapy through use of a rapid microarray assay on blood cultures positive for Enterococcus species. J Clin Microbiol 2013;51(12):4008–11.

63. Nicolsen NC, LeCroy N, Alby K, et al. Clinical outcomes with rapid detection of methicillin-resistant and methicillin-susceptible Staphylococcus aureus isolates from routine blood cultures. J Clin Microbiol 2013;51(12):4126–9.

64. Wong JR, Bauer KA, Mangino JE, et al. Antimicrobial stewardship pharmacist interventions for coagulase-negative staphylococci positive blood cultures using rapid polymerase chain reaction. Ann Pharmacother 2012;46(11):1484–90.

65. Altobelli E, Mohan R, Mach KE, et al. Integrated biosensor assay for rapid uropathogen identification and phenotypic antimicrobial susceptibility testing. Eur Urol Focus 2017;3(2–3):293–9.

66. Sundqvist M, Olafsson J, Matuschek E. EUCAST breakpoints can be used to interpret direct susceptibility testing of Enterobacteriaceae from urine samples. APMIS 2015;123(2):152–5.

67. Coorevits L, Boelens J, Claeys G. Direct susceptibility testing by disk diffusion on clinical samples: a rapid and accurate tool for antibiotic stewardship. Eur J Clin Microbiol Infect Dis 2015;34(6):1207–12.

68. Ilki A, Bekdemir P, Ulger N, et al. Rapid reporting of urine culture results: impact of the uro-quick screening system. New Microbiol 2010;33(2):147–53.

69. Ivancic V, Mastali M, Percy N, et al. Rapid antimicrobial susceptibility determination of uropathogens in clinical urine specimens by use of ATP bioluminescence. J Clin Microbiol 2008;46(4):1213–9.

70. Breteler KB, Rentenaar RJ, Verkaart G, et al. Performance and clinical significance of direct antimicrobial susceptibility testing on urine from hospitalized patients. Scand J Infect Dis 2011;43(10):771–6.

71. Moreno LZ, Matajira CEC, Poor AP, et al. Identification through MALDI-TOF mass spectrometry and antimicrobial susceptibility profiling of bacterial pathogens isolated from sow urinary tract infection. Vet Q 2018;38(1):1–8.

72. Depret F, Aubry A, Fournier A, et al. Beta LACTA testing may not improve treatment decisions made with MALDI-TOF MS-informed antimicrobial stewardship advice for patients with Gram-negative bacteraemia: a prospective comparative study. J Med Microbiol 2018;67(2):183–9.

73. Tre-Hardy M, Lambert B, Despas N, et al. MALDI-TOF MS identification and antimicrobial susceptibility testing directly from positive enrichment broth. J Microbiol Methods 2017;141:32–4.

74. Maxson T, Taylor-Howell CL, Minogue TD. Semi-quantitative MALDI-TOF for antimicrobial susceptibility testing in Staphylococcus aureus. PloS One 2017;12(8): e0183899.

75. Verroken A, Defourny L, le Polain de Waroux O, et al. Correction: clinical impact of MALDI-TOF MS identification and rapid susceptibility testing on adequate antimicrobial treatment in sepsis with positive blood cultures. PloS One 2016; 11(9):e0160537.

76. Fitzgerald C, Stapleton P, Phelan E, et al. Rapid identification and antimicrobial susceptibility testing of positive blood cultures using MALDI-TOF MS and a modification of the standardised disc diffusion test: a pilot study. J Clin Pathol 2016. https://doi.org/10.1136/jclinpath-2015-203436.

77. Machen A, Drake T, Wang YF. Same day identification and full panel antimicrobial susceptibility testing of bacteria from positive blood culture bottles made possible by a combined lysis-filtration method with MALDI-TOF VITEK mass spectrometry and the VITEK2 system. PloS One 2014;9(2):e87870.

78. O'Donnell LA, Guarascio AJ. The intersection of antimicrobial stewardship and microbiology: educating the next generation of health care professionals. FEMS Microbiol Lett 2017;364(1) [pii:fnw281].

79. Snyder JW, Munier GK, Johnson CL. Comparison of the BD GeneOhm methicillin-resistant Staphylococcus aureus (MRSA) PCR assay to culture by use of BBL CHROMagar MRSA for detection of MRSA in nasal surveillance cultures from intensive care unit patients. J Clin Microbiol 2010;48(4):1305–9.

80. Peterson LR, Liesenfeld O, Woods CW, et al. Multicenter evaluation of the Light-Cycler methicillin-resistant Staphylococcus aureus (MRSA) advanced test as a rapid method for detection of MRSA in nasal surveillance swabs. J Clin Microbiol 2010;48(5):1661–6.

81. Paule SM, Mehta M, Hacek DM, et al. Chromogenic media vs real-time PCR for nasal surveillance of methicillin-resistant Staphylococcus aureus: impact on detection of MRSA-positive persons. Am J Clin Pathol 2009;131(4):532–9.

82. Munoz P, Hortal J, Giannella M, et al. Nasal carriage of S. aureus increases the risk of surgical site infection after major heart surgery. J Hosp Infect 2008;68(1): 25–31.

83. Schweizer ML, Chiang HY, Septimus E, et al. Association of a bundled intervention with surgical site infections among patients undergoing cardiac, hip, or knee surgery. JAMA 2015;313(21):2162–71.

84. Bebko SP, Green DM, Awad SS. Effect of a preoperative decontamination protocol on surgical site infections in patients undergoing elective orthopedic surgery with hardware implantation. JAMA Surg 2015;150(5):390–5.

85. Norton TD, Skeete F, Dubrovskaya Y, et al. Orthopedic surgical site infections: analysis of causative bacteria and implications for antibiotic stewardship. Am J Orthop (Belle Mead NJ) 2014;43(5):E89–92.

86. Geladari A, Karampatakis T, Antachopoulos C, et al. Epidemiological surveillance of multidrug-resistant gram-negative bacteria in a solid organ transplantation department. Transpl Infect Dis 2017;19(3). https://doi.org/10.1111/tid. 12686.

87. Demiraslan H, Cevahir F, Berk E, et al. Is surveillance for colonization of carbapenem-resistant gram-negative bacteria important in adult bone marrow transplantation units? Am J Infect Control 2017;45(7):735–9.

88. Giuffre M, Geraci DM, Bonura C, et al. The increasing challenge of multidrug-resistant gram-negative bacilli: results of a 5-year active surveillance program in a neonatal intensive care unit. Medicine 2016;95(10):e3016.

89. Freeman R, Ironmonger D, Puleston R, et al. Enhanced surveillance of carbapenemase-producing Gram-negative bacteria to support national and international prevention and control efforts. Clin Microbiol Infect 2016;22(10): 896–7.

90. Maechler F, Pena Diaz LA, Schroder C, et al. Prevalence of carbapenem-resistant organisms and other Gram-negative MDRO in German ICUs: first results from the national nosocomial infection surveillance system (KISS). Infection 2015;43(2):163–8.

91. Mataseje LF, Bryce E, Roscoe D, et al. Carbapenem-resistant Gram-negative bacilli in Canada 2009-10: results from the Canadian nosocomial infection surveillance program (CNISP). J Antimicrob Chemother 2012; 67(6):1359–67.

92. Bertrand X, Dowzicky MJ. Antimicrobial susceptibility among gram-negative isolates collected from intensive care units in North America, Europe, the Asia-Pacific Rim, Latin America, the Middle East, and Africa between 2004 and 2009 as part of the Tigecycline Evaluation and Surveillance Trial. Clin Ther 2012;34(1):124–37.

93. Parm U, Metsvaht T, Sepp E, et al. Mucosal surveillance cultures in predicting Gram-negative late-onset sepsis in neonatal intensive care units. J Hosp Infect 2011;78(4):327–32.

94. Krutova M, Kinross P, Barbut F, et al. How to: surveillance of Clostridium difficile infections. Clin Microbiol Infect 2018;24(5):469–75.

95. Guh AY, McDonald LC. Active surveillance and isolation of asymptomatic carriers of Clostridium difficile at hospital admission: containing what lies under the waterline. JAMA Intern Med 2016;176(6):805–6.

96. Le Saux N, Gravel D, Mulvey M, et al. Healthcare-associated Clostridium difficile infections and strain diversity in pediatric hospitals in the canadian nosocomial infection surveillance program, 2007-2011. J Pediatric Infect Dis Soc 2015;4(4): e151–4.

97. Berrington A. Impact of mandatory Clostridium difficile surveillance on diagnostic services. J Hosp Infect 2004;58(3):241–2.

98. Timsit JF, Azoulay E, Schwebel C, et al. Empirical micafungin treatment and survival without invasive fungal infection in adults with ICU-acquired sepsis, candida colonization, and multiple organ failure: the EMPIRICUS randomized clinical trial. JAMA 2016;316(15):1555–64.

99. Giannella M, Rodriguez-Sanchez B, Roa PL, et al. Should lower respiratory tract secretions from intensive care patients be systematically screened for influenza virus during the influenza season? Crit Care 2012;16(3):R104.

100. Ha J, Hong SK, Han GH, et al. Same-day identification and antimicrobial susceptibility testing of bacteria in positive blood culture broths using short-term incubation on solid medium with the MicroFlex LT, Vitek-MS, and Vitek2 systems. Ann Lab Med 2018;38(3):235–41.

101. Li C, Ding S, Huang Y, et al. Detection of AmpC beta-Lactamase-producing Gram-negative bacteria by MALDI-TOF MS analysis. J Hosp Infect 2017. https://doi.org/10.1016/j.jhin.2017.11.010.

102. Canali C, Spillum E, Valvik M, et al. Real-time digital bright field technology for rapid antibiotic susceptibility testing. Methods Mol Biol 2018;1736:75–84.

103. Syal K, Shen S, Yang Y, et al. Rapid antibiotic susceptibility testing of uropathogenic E. coli by tracking submicron scale motion of single bacterial cells. ACS Sens 2017;2(8):1231–9.

104. Schoepp NG, Schlappi TS, Curtis MS, et al. Rapid pathogen-specific phenotypic antibiotic susceptibility testing using digital LAMP quantification in clinical samples. Sci Transl Med 2017;9(410) [pii:eaal3693].

105. Hombach M, Jetter M, Keller PM, et al. Rapid detection of ESBL, carbapenemases, MRSA and other important resistance phenotypes within 6-8 h by automated disc diffusion antibiotic susceptibility testing. J Antimicrob Chemother 2017;72(11):3063–9.

106. Abbasi J. Rapid test for antibiotic susceptibility. JAMA 2017;318(14):1314.

107. Liu CY, Han YY, Shih PH, et al. Rapid bacterial antibiotic susceptibility test based on simple surface-enhanced Raman spectroscopic biomarkers. Sci Rep 2016;6:23375.

108. Le Page S, Dubourg G, Rolain JM. Evaluation of the Scan(R) 1200 as a rapid tool for reading antibiotic susceptibility testing by the disc diffusion technique. J Antimicrob Chemother 2016;71(12):3424–31.

109. Mezger A, Gullberg E, Goransson J, et al. A general method for rapid determination of antibiotic susceptibility and species in bacterial infections. J Clin Microbiol 2015;53(2):425–32.

110. Le Page S, Raoult D, Rolain JM. Real-time video imaging as a new and rapid tool for antibiotic susceptibility testing by the disc diffusion method: a paradigm for evaluating resistance to imipenem and identifying extended-spectrum beta-lactamases. Int J Antimicrob Agents 2015;45(1):61–5.

111. Huang TH, Ning X, Wang X, et al. Rapid cytometric antibiotic susceptibility testing utilizing adaptive multidimensional statistical metrics. Anal Chem 2015; 87(3):1941–9.

112. He J, Mu X, Guo Z, et al. A novel microbead-based microfluidic device for rapid bacterial identification and antibiotic susceptibility testing. Eur J Clin Microbiol Infect Dis 2014;33(12):2223–30.

113. Erdem SS, Khan S, Palanisami A, et al. Rapid, low-cost fluorescent assay of beta-lactamase-derived antibiotic resistance and related antibiotic susceptibility. J Biomed Opt 2014;19(10):105007.

114. Maurer FP, Christner M, Hentschke M, et al. Advances in rapid identification and susceptibility testing of bacteria in the clinical microbiology laboratory: implications for patient care and antimicrobial stewardship programs. Infect Dis Rep 2017;9(1):6839.

115. MacKenzie FM, Gould IM, Bruce J, et al. The role of microbiology and pharmacy departments in the stewardship of antibiotic prescribing in European hospitals. J Hosp Infect 2007;65(Suppl 2):73–81.

116. Moehring RW, Anderson DJ. Antimicrobial stewardship as part of the infection prevention effort. Curr Infect Dis Rep 2012;14(6):592–600.

117. Tonna AP, Gould IM, Stewart D. A cross-sectional survey of antimicrobial stewardship strategies in UK hospitals. J Clin Pharm Ther 2014;39(5):516–20.

118. Guillard P, de La Blanchardiere A, Cattoir V, et al. Antimicrobial stewardship and linezolid. Int J Clin Pharm 2014;36(5):1059–68.

119. Forrest GN, Van Schooneveld TC, Kullar R, et al. Use of electronic health records and clinical decision support systems for antimicrobial stewardship. Clin Infect Dis 2014;59(Suppl 3):S122–33.

120. Borde JP, Litterst S, Ruhnke M, et al. Implementing an intensified antibiotic stewardship programme targeting cephalosporin and fluoroquinolone use in a 200-bed community hospital in Germany. Infection 2015;43(1):45–50.

121. Dekmezian M, Beal SG, Damashek MJ, et al. The SUCCESS model for laboratory performance and execution of rapid molecular diagnostics in patients with sepsis. Proc (Bayl Univ Med Cent) 2015;28(2):144–50.

122. Munoz P, Valerio M, Vena A, et al. Antifungal stewardship in daily practice and health economic implications. Mycoses 2015;58(Suppl 2):14–25.

123. Barlam TF, Cosgrove SE, Abbo LM, et al. Implementing an antibiotic stewardship program: guidelines by the infectious diseases society of America and the Society for Healthcare Epidemiology of America. Clin Infect Dis 2016; 62(10):e51–77.

124. Barlam TF, Cosgrove SE, Abbo LM, et al. Executive summary: implementing an antibiotic stewardship program: guidelines by the infectious diseases society of America and the society for healthcare epidemiology of America. Clin Infect Dis 2016;62(10):1197–202.

125. Lipsky BA, Dryden M, Gottrup F, et al. Antimicrobial stewardship in wound care: a position paper from the British Society for antimicrobial chemotherapy and European Wound Management Association. J Antimicrob Chemother 2016;71(11): 3026–35.

126. Goff DA, Karam GH, Haines ST. Impact of a national antimicrobial stewardship mentoring program: insights and lessons learned. Am J Health Syst Pharm 2017;74(4):224–31.

127. Inacio J, Barnes LM, Jeffs S, et al. Master of Pharmacy students' knowledge and awareness of antibiotic use, resistance and stewardship. Curr Pharm Teach Learn 2017;9(4):551–9.

128. Geiger K, Brown J. Rapid testing for methicillin-resistant Staphylococcus aureus: implications for antimicrobial stewardship. Am J Health Syst Pharm 2013;70(4):335–42.

129. Lowman W. Key to antimicrobial stewardship success: surveillance by diagnostic microbiology laboratories. S Afr Med J 2015;105(5):359–60.

Current and Future Opportunities for Rapid Diagnostics in Antimicrobial Stewardship

Tristan T. Timbrook, PharmD, MBA[a], Emily S. Spivak, MD, MHS[b],
Kimberly E. Hanson, MD, MHS[b,c,d,*]

KEYWORDS

- Antimicrobial stewardship • Rapid diagnostics • Diagnostic stewardship • Infections

KEY POINTS

- Rapid diagnostic testing has greatly affected the landscape of antimicrobial stewardship programs and, in many instances, is associated with improved patient care.
- Antimicrobial stewardship intervention is required to fully realize the potential clinical impact of rapid testing for bloodstream infections. Whether the same benefits can be achieved for other infectious diseases requires additional research.
- Partnership between the clinical microbiology laboratory and antimicrobial stewardship programs is expected to become increasingly important as new and more complicated tests as well as novel diagnostic approaches become available in the future.

INTRODUCTION

Rapid microbiology diagnostics have consistently been shown to decrease time to organism identification and thus, potentially enable earlier initiation of targeted antimicrobial therapy.[1,2] Optimizing and minimizing unnecessary antimicrobial use is imperative in the age of increasing rates of *Clostridium difficile* infection (CDI), antimicrobial-resistant infections, and antimicrobial-related adverse drug events.

Disclosure statement: T.T. Timbrook has served as a speaker and/or advisor for BioFire Diagnostics, GenMark Diagnostics, and Roche Diagnostics. K.E. Hanson has multiple investigator initiated studies with BioFire Diagnostics. E.S. Spivak has no potential conflicts of interest.
[a] Department of Pharmacy, University of Utah, 50 North Medical Drive, Salt Lake City, UT 84132, USA; [b] Department of Medicine, University of Utah, 30 North 1900 East, Salt Lake City, UT 84132, USA; [c] Institute for Clinical and Experimental Pathology, ARUP Laboratories, 500 Chipeta Way, Salt Lake City, UT 84108, USA; [d] Department of Pathology, University of Utah, 15 North Medical Drive East, Salt Lake City, UT 84112, USA
* Corresponding author. School of Medicine, University of Utah, 30 North 1900 East, Room 4B319, Salt Lake City, UT 84132.
E-mail address: kim.hanson@hsc.utah.edu

Med Clin N Am 102 (2018) 899–911
https://doi.org/10.1016/j.mcna.2018.05.004
0025-7125/18/© 2018 Elsevier Inc. All rights reserved.

medical.theclinics.com

Significant advances in clinical microbiology diagnostics have been made over the last decade. A wide array of advanced methods with rapid turnaround times and the ability to detect multiple pathogens with high sensitivity have become available. However, many of these new technologies are expensive and few studies have established cost-effectiveness and/or best implementation strategies to maximize value.

Antimicrobial stewardship is a multidisciplinary program of activities that optimizes antimicrobial use to improve clinical outcomes and minimize unintended consequences of antimicrobial misuse. In collaboration with the clinical microbiology laboratory, stewardship teams are playing an increasingly important role in guiding best use of rapid diagnostic testing (RDT). Recent Infectious Diseases Society of America guidelines for implementing an Antimicrobial Stewardship Program (ASP) recommend ASPs advocate for RDT for respiratory infections and bloodstream infections (BSIs) as a means to improve antimicrobial use.[3] The rapid respiratory viral testing has the potential to reduce inappropriate antibiotic use; however, the potential impacts of respiratory viral testing to date have been mixed and the addition of active ASP intervention may improve results. Because the use of RDT for BSIs in the absence of active ASP intervention has not been shown to consistently improve antimicrobial use, guidelines specifically recommend the use of RDT for BSI only if paired with active ASP support and interpretation to providers.[3–6] Active ASP intervention can take on many forms and include activities beyond treatment recommendations; however, proper implementation is labor and resource intensive. With regulatory requirements leading to expansion of ASPs across all health care settings, further understanding of the clinical impact that ASP interventions can have when paired with rapid diagnostic capabilities is imperative for resource allocation.

Although not exhaustive in scope, this review focuses on rapid diagnostic modalities available for bacterial BSIs, candidemia, respiratory tract infections, and gastrointestinal (GI) infections. Specifically, we highlight what is known about the most effective application of these diagnostics in clinical settings, focusing on their clinical utility, cost-effectiveness, and interplay with antimicrobial stewardship efforts.

BLOODSTREAM INFECTIONS
Bacterial

Several US Food and Drug Administration (FDA)–approved RDTs are commercially available for the diagnosis of BSI. Current tests for bacteria are designed to be applied to aliquots from positive blood culture bottles and detect only the most common (>80%) causes of BSI. Available assays are based on peptide nucleic acid fluorescent in situ hybridization (PNA-FISH) with or without digital microscopy, polymerase chain reaction (PCR), or different forms of nanoparticle array technology (**Table 1**). In addition to organism identification, some of the PCR and array-based platforms also provide limited genotypic resistance information. The Accelerate Pheno system (Accelerate Diagnostics, Tucson, AZ, USA) is unique in that it combines organism identification using FISH probes with rapid phenotypic susceptibility results.[7] In addition to RDT applied to blood culture aliquots, 2 matrix-assisted laser desorption/ionization-time of flight (MALDI-TOF) mass spectroscopy platforms are FDA approved for the rapid identification of organisms in pure culture. Faster time to organism identification and information on resistance yields opportunities for clinicians to target antimicrobial therapy in a more rapid manner, which can translate into improved clinical outcomes. However, an important limitation of all current technologies is the inability to accurately analyze polymicrobial cultures and a dearth of assays capable of detecting resistance in Gram-negative organisms.

Table 1
Food and Drug Administration–approved rapid diagnostic tests supported by clinical outcomes data for bloodstream infections, respiratory tract infections, and gastrointestinal tract infections

Technology	Manufacturer, System	Syndrome Testing	Targets	Time to Result (h)
PNA-FISH	AdvanDx, PNA-FISH Accelerate PhenoTest; PNA-FISH with morphokinetic cellular analysis	Blood	1–15	0.3–1.5 for ID 7 for susceptibility
Limited target PCR or LAMP	GeneOhm, StaphSR	Blood	1	2
	Cepheid, Xpert MRSA/SA BC	Blood	1	1
	BD MAX	GI	4	3
	Prodesse	GI, Respiratory	3–4	3–4
	Meridian Bioscience, Illumigene	GI (*Clostridium difficile* only)	1	1
	BD GeneOhm, Cdiff Assay	GI (*C difficile* only)	1	2
	Cepheid, Xpert *C difficile*	GI (*C difficile* only)	1–2	0.5
MALDI-TOF	bioMerieux, MALDI-TOF	Any	Multitude of bacterial and fungal organisms in pure culture	0.5
	Brucker, MALDI-TOF	Any	Multitude of bacterial and fungal organisms in pure culture	0.5
Multiplex array panel	BioFire, FilmArray	Blood, GI, Respiratory	14–27	1
	Nanosphere, Verigene	Blood, GI, Respiratory	1–16	2
	Luminex, xTAG	GI, Respiratory	9–20	5–8
NMR	T2 Biosystems, T2Candida	Whole blood	3	3–5

Abbreviations: LAMP, loop-mediated isothermal amplification; MALDI-TOF, matrix-assisted laser desorption/ionization-time of flight; NMR, nuclear magnetic resonance.

Most outcomes studies evaluating the impact of RDTs combined with ASPs in BSI have been quasi-experimental and have focused on PNA-FISH, multiplex PCR, or MALDI-TOF. Early evaluations of PNA-FISH combined with ASP intervention found significant decreases in length of stay (LOS) for patients with blood cultures growing coagulase-negative Staphylococci and decreases in time to effective therapy and mortality among enterococcal bacteremia.[1,8] Subsequently, limited target PCR panels along with active stewardship have demonstrated decreases in time to optimal therapy, LOS, and hospital costs among *Staphylococcus aureus* bacteremia patients.[9] Thereafter, MALDI-TOF along with ASP intervention demonstrated decreased time to effective therapy, optimal therapy, LOS, and hospital costs per patient.[10,11] Lastly, multiplex panel testing and ASPs have shown significantly decreased time to effective therapy among vancomycin-resistant *Enterococcus* and extended-spectrum beta-lactamase BSIs by more than a day.[12,13] Conversely, in the absence of ASPs, RDTs in BSI have demonstrated a lack of clinical impact.[4–6]

Two randomized control trials (RCTs) evaluating the impact of RDT for BSI have been performed. One trial evaluated the impact of a multiplex PCR platform that detects bacteria, fungi, and resistance markers from positive blood cultures on patient outcomes.[2] Patients were divided into 3 arms: standard of care, multiplex PCR testing with templated comments issued in the microbiology results report, or multiplex PCR testing with templated comments plus real-time prospective audit and feedback by an ASP. Decreases in broad spectrum antimicrobial use were noted among both experimental groups versus the control. Time to de-escalation was most pronounced among the active stewardship intervention arm compared with the control group (21 h vs 34 h, P<.001). The study did not show a decrease in LOS, mortality, or cost, although the authors note that the study was not powered to detect these differences. Another BSI RCT with MALDI-TOF testing in both arms randomized real-time stewardship review of MALDI-TOF results and feedback of antimicrobial recommendations to providers and noted significant differences in time to both active and appropriate therapy among ASP intervention patients.[14]

Individual observational studies have had mixed results, possibly highlighting differences in technologies, patient populations, implementation strategies, local epidemiology of resistance, local empirical prescribing practices and limited sample sizes. However, meta-analysis data also suggest RDTs for BSI have an impact on time to effective therapy, mortality, and LOS when coupled with ASP.[15]

Few studies have performed cost analyses of RDT and ASP implementation in BSI.[16] One study evaluated the cost of MALDI-TOF with ASP intervention in BSIs, including fixed direct, variable direct, and fixed indirect costs from 13 cost centers. Including the cost of the ASP pharmacist review and increased laboratory costs, average total hospitalization cost per patient was reduced by nearly $2500 (P = nonsignificant [NS]).[17] Moreover, PCR testing in S aureus BSIs and active ASP review and intervention in BSIs have both been demonstrated as the dominant strategies as compared with the standard of care in cost-effectiveness studies.[18] Aside from these studies, robust cost-effectiveness evaluations of ASPs and RDTs in BSI are lacking, and more data are needed to better understand the clinical and financial impact of these tests and inform stewardship efforts and resource allocation.

Fungal/Candida

For patients with candidemia, FDA-approved RDTs include PNA-FISH, multiplex PCR panels, Accelerate Pheno, and MALDI-TOF. Assays differ in the number of Candida species detected; otherwise the use and turnaround time of these technologies mirror those for bacterial BSIs. In contrast, the T2Candida (T2Biosystems, Lexington, MA, USA) assay is a new paradigm in that testing is performed directly on whole blood from patients with suspected candidemia. T2Candida uses a magnetic resonance technology to achieve sensitivity on par with blood culture within 3 to 5 hours as opposed to incubated cultures that take days to become positive.[19] All of these technologies have the potential to decrease time to effective therapy among patients with candidemia, and early treatment is associated with decreases in mortality.[20,21]

Literature specific to RDT and ASPs in candidemia remains limited. An early PNA-FISH study reflected possible cost avoidance for antifungals in candidemias.[22] Another study looked at the implementation of ASP intervention and PNA-FISH on candidemia patient clinical outcomes. Time to targeted therapy was significantly decreased along with decreased average cost of $415 per patient.[23] Similarly, a subgroup of candidemia patients from a large MALD-TOF with active ASP study reflected a trend to decreased time to effective therapy (difference of 23 h, P=NS) and decreased mortality (33.3% vs 17.7%, P=NS).

To date, data on clinical outcomes associated with T2Candida and ASPs remain limited.[19] A recent quasi-experimental multi-center study evaluated the impact of T2Candida implementation with ASP review as compared with standard of care with routine blood cultures on clinical outcomes. Investigators found a difference in median time to appropriate antifungal therapy of 17 hours (P=.003) and no difference in LOS or mortality. Fewer cases of *Candida* eye involvement were noted among the postimplementation group (odds ratio 0.40, P=.028), possibly related to earlier effective therapy from the T2Candida identification.

Cost analysis of the use of RDTs among ASPs in candidemia has suggested possible cost savings from decreased echinocandin use.[22,23] Although the single study evaluating T2Candida with ASP intervention did not perform a cost analysis, cost-effectiveness analyses of T2Candida have suggested a high dependence of benefit on candida bloodstream prevalence coupled with the ability to withhold or stop antifungal therapy in patients with low-to-moderate risk of candidemia.[24,25]

RESPIRATORY TRACT INFECTIONS

Streptococcus pneumoniae and *Legionella pneumophila* urinary antigens, along with influenza enzyme immunosorbent assays (EIAs) and PCR, have historically been used by clinicians and stewardship programs alike to rapidly target optimal care to patients with respiratory tract infections. More recently, multiplex panels have emerged to allow for detection of a multitude of virus targets in as little as 1 to 2 hours.

Although data specific to the use of multiplex respiratory viral panels in conjunction with ASPs remain largely absent, several studies give insight into the use of these technologies to achieve stewardship principles. An open-label RCT evaluated the use of a molecular point-of-care multiplex respiratory testing (POCT) versus standard of care testing among emergency department and acute medical unit adults, notably in the absence of any antimicrobial stewardship interventions.[26] Similar numbers of patients received antibiotics (84% POCT group and 83% among controls, P=.84). Although the mean duration of antibiotics did not differ between groups, more POCT patients had either single doses or short courses of less than 48 hours compared with control patients (17% vs 9%, P=.0047). POCT was also associated with decreased LOS, more appropriate antiviral treatment of influenza, and shorter average durations of antibiotics among patients with asthma and chronic obstructive pulmonary disease. Similarly, observational data have demonstrated benefits of multiplex respiratory testing in clinical management of patients, although the impact has been limited to patients with influenza. One study using multivariate regression showed that only multiplex respiratory testing diagnosis of influenza positive results was associated with lower odds of admission, LOS, duration of antibiotics, and number of imaging studies obtained, whereas detection of other viruses did not change clinical management including use of antibiotics.[27] Similar differences in clinical management of influenza and noninfluenza virus patients has been shown in other studies, which reflected less antibiotic use among influenza positive patients but had no impact on antibiotic use among noninfluenza virus patients.[28,29]

In summary, the rapid identification of respiratory viruses yields the opportunity for antibiotic avoidance. However, reduction in unnecessary antibiotic use has not been consistently observed across studies especially for adult patients and when detecting viruses other than influenza. The main limitation of current respiratory molecular panels is a lack of bacterial targets for community- or hospital-acquired pneumonia.

Without added confidence that a patient with pneumonia does not have a bacterial infection, clinicians may be reluctant to withhold antibiotics even when a respiratory virus is detected. Furthermore, real-time stewardship of testing performed near the patient in the ED or outpatient clinic is logistically difficult and potentially resource intense. Because a significant proportion of inappropriate antibiotic use occurs for viral upper respiratory tract infections in outpatient setting,[30] this may be one area for ASPs to focus effort in the future.

The use of procalcitonin (PCT) in patients with acute respiratory infections has also been shown to decrease in mortality, duration of antibiotic exposure, and antibiotic-related side effects.[31] Although PCT is often used by ASPs and is recommend by ASP guidelines, data on active stewardship interventions around PCT are limited.[3] Another possible approach toward increased pragmatic antibiotic use among patients with viral respiratory tract infection has been suggested using the combination of multiplex respiratory panel and PCT testing. A pilot RCT of this approach combined with an algorithm for interpretation for providers resulted in less patients receiving antibiotics on discharge among patients with low PCT level and who are viral positive in addition to shorter durations of antibiotics among multiplex viral panel and PCT-tested patients whose providers adhered to the algorithm versus standard of care patients. Real-world experience suggests that the combination of multiplex viral panel testing and PCT without concomitant interpretive algorithms have minimal impact on antibiotic use, again highlighting the need for interpretive guidelines at minimum and possibly results paired with active stewardship interventions in order to maximize impacts on antibiotic prescribing.[32]

Beyond multiplex PCR and PCT testing in respiratory illness, another RDT used by ASPs to optimize patient management has been the use of screening for nasal methicillin-resistant *S aureus* (MRSA) colonization for vancomycin de-escalation in suspected MRSA pneumonia. Meta-analysis data suggest a low positive predictive value and therefore limited utility in diagnosing MRSA pneumonia.[33] However, the negative predictive value ranges from 95% to 98%, effectively ruling out MRSA pneumonia and translating into either the avoidance or the discontinuation of anti-MRSA therapies such as vancomycin. An ASP using this approach to de-escalate vancomycin among intensive care unit patients during a 2-year period observed an average cost avoidance of $108 per patient based on the cost of vancomycin, vancomycin laboratory levels, and surveillance testing.[34] Further implementation data suggest a median reduction of vancomycin by 2.1 days of therapy per patient ($P<.0001$).[35]

GASTROINTESTINAL TRACT INFECTIONS

Akin to BSI and respiratory syndromic testing, molecular GI panels have emerged to allow for a multitude of targets to be tested with results back in about 1 to 2 hours. Moreover, in recent years, *C difficile* testing has changed from moderate sensitivity EIA to highly sensitive PCR testing as the standard of care. With this change some institutions have seen their CDI rates double with PCR.[36] ASPs have worked hand in hand with infection control, microbiology, and information technology departments to mitigate these issues and improve diagnostic stewardship.

Clostridium difficile

As CDI rates are often a chosen metric for the performance of ASPs, ensuring optimal testing of the correct patient to avoid incorrect diagnosis remains a paramount goal for ASPs. Several studies have attempted to address this issue by focusing on selecting the right patient for testing or increasing the pretest probability of true disease.

Approaches to this have included enforcing testing criteria to greater than or equal to 3 unformed stools in 24 hours and absence of laxative use in prior 48 hours, resulting in significant decreases in inappropriate testing.[37] In addition to evidence of inappropriate testing in setting of laxative use, other data have shown half of the patients with positive CDI testing having laxatives continued more than 24 hours after the positive test and treatment is often not in accordance with guidelines.[38] These data highlight the opportunity for infection prevention, ASPs, and microbiology to collaborate in order to improve *C difficile* testing and management.[39]

Some studies have analyzed the effect of real-time stewardship coupled with CDI RDT. One study looked at the impact of an ASP CDI bundle consisting of ensuring appropriate CDI therapy based on severity, discontinuation of concomitant antimicrobials and acid suppressants when possible, and consultation of infectious diseases and/or surgery in severe CDI or severe complicated CDI.[40] The ASP received real-time notification of positive CDI results. Bundle compliance improved overall through ASP intervention (81% vs 45%, $P<.001$) with adherence with individual components improving through ASP intervention including discontinuation of acid suppressants (90% vs 18%, $P<.001$) and administration of appropriate CDI therapy based on severity (82% vs 64%, $P<.009$). Similar data on CDI RDT coupled with real-time ASP notification and intervention have reflected decrease in time to initiation of CDI therapy, improved adherence to standards of care, and discontinuation of acid suppressants.[41–43]

Polymerase chain reaction panels
Clinical outcomes data on multiplex GI panels for diagnosis of diarrhea have been limited. While an RCT of GI panels is currently underway, the existing outcomes data are limited to retrospective studies.[44–46] A retrospective observational study compared patient management and outcomes among patients receiving standard of care versus multiplex GI testing.[44] Patients with multiplex testing received less antibiotics (1.73 days vs 2.12, $P=.06$), fewer imaging studies ($P=.0002$), and decreased average time from stool collection to patient discharge (3.4 vs 3.9 days, $P=.04$). Similarly, other retrospective data have suggested that multiplex GI panels can have an impact on clinical management and antibiotic use that can likely be augmented by active ASP intervention.[45] To date, data evaluating active stewardship intervention paired with multiplex GI panels are lacking. Cost-effectiveness data have suggested potential improvements in laboratory workflow and organism detection rates while achieving cost-effectiveness through decreased contact isolation requirements.[47]

RAPID DIAGNOSTIC TEST IMPLEMENTATION CONSIDERATIONS

As suggested by many of the aforementioned studies, RDTs generally require facilitation by ASPs to ensure timely clinical intervention and maximize the impact of these technologies.[15] A recent study highlighted this requirement by evaluating the performance of clinicians interpreting mock RDT results in BSI at an institution with previous education sessions, guidance, and a clinical pathway on their stewardship Web site for the RDT.[48] Of the 156 respondents, cases were misinterpreted 14% to 82% of the time. Clearly, adequate stewardship resources to monitor and yield feedback to frontline clinicians, preferably in real-time, is needed. Moreover, data reflect not only that this is needed but also that providers appreciate unsolicited interventions and recommendations from ASPs on RDT results.[49] To achieve the goal of optimal RDT implementation, it may be beneficial to form a Diagnostics Committee, similar to a Pharmacy and Therapeutics Committee, where key stakeholders can strategize together to determine what diagnostic assays would best meet the needs of clinicians and how best to incorporate them into clinical workflow while ensuring optimal patient outcomes, cost-effectiveness, and diagnostic stewardship.[50] Collaborative justification of these new technologies by microbiology and ASPs to administration can be made, with proposals highlighting improved laboratory workflow, compliance with Centers for Disease Control and Prevention core elements of hospital ASPs and other regulatory requirements (**Box 1**), cost-effectiveness data, and reductions in LOS.[51]

FUTURE DIRECTIONS

Rapid tests for bloodstream, respiratory, and GI infections have helped to revolutionize the practice of clinical microbiology, but major unmet diagnostic needs remain for these diseases. Current RDTs are limited in their ability to accurately determine which patients have an infection requiring antibiotics and if a patient is infected, what drug or combination of drugs are expected to be most effective and least toxic. Although a comprehensive review of emerging technologies for microbiology is beyond the scope of this review, several new assays for BSI or lower respiratory tract infection (LRTI) have been developed and are either completing clinical trials to support review by the FDA or have been submitted to the FDA as an in vitro diagnostic device.

Time is of the essence especially in the management of severe sepsis and septic shock. Current guidelines recommend initiating broad-spectrum antibiotics within the first hour of recognition of shock,[52] but approximately 20% of patients receive

---

Box 1
Compliance with Centers for Disease Control and Prevention core elements of hospital antibiotic stewardship programs through the use of RDTs

- Leadership support
  - Financial commitment to support microbiology and stewardship for RDT implementation
- Accountability for program by physician leader
  - Physician leader ensures optimal implementation of RDT into clinical practice (eg, clinical pathways) to achieve improvement in outcomes
- Drug expertise by pharmacist leader for improving antibiotic use
  - Responsible for daily prospective audit and feedback on RDT results for optimizing antibiotic use
- Actions on specific interventions to improve antibiotic use
  - Routine interventions around specific RDT, such as blood cultures, can be implemented to improve certain infectious syndrome-specific antibiotic use
- Tracking and monitoring
  - Multiple metrics for optimal use of RDT can be evaluated, including adherence to clinical pathways or guidelines, acceptance of recommendations, and durations of therapy
- Reporting information to staff on improving antibiotic use
  - Metrics of RDT-specific interventions shared with key stakeholders; appropriate diagnostics usage report card shared with front line providers
- Education to providers
  - Instruct clinicians both during RDT implementation and when providing feedback on RDT use during daily clinical activities

Abbreviation: RDT, rapid diagnostic test.
Adapted from Centers for Disease Control and Prevention (CDC). Core elements of hospital antibiotic stewardship programs. Available at: https://www.cdc.gov/antibiotic-use/healthcare/implementation/core-elements.html. Accessed May 1, 2018.

ineffective empirical treatment.[53] Inappropriate initial therapy is associated with poor patient outcomes. Current BSI assays require preamplification of organisms in culture for hours or days to have enough sensitivity to accurately detect targeted bacteria. Thus, these tests are only useful for modifying empirical treatment after several doses have been administered. As described earlier for *Candida*, T2 technology enables direct detection in blood, significantly reducing time to organism identification. T2Biosystems has developed a bacterial panel, which was submitted to the FDA for 510(k) premarket review in September of 2017.[54] The assay detects and differentiates *Escherichia coli*, *Klebsiella pneumoniae*, *Pseudomonas aeruginosa*, *Acinetobacter baumannii*, *S aureus*, and *Enterococcus faecium*. Although the panel is limited in the breadth of organisms it identifies, the test may enable more rapid alterations in empirical therapy to include coverage of drug-resistant species based on local prevalence and antibiograms as well as faster time to de-escalation of empirical broad-spectrum therapy. Clearly, more information on whether the organisms detected actually harbor resistance determinants would be preferred for optimal antibiotic prescribing. Other novel methods for direct organism detection with simultaneous assessment of antibiotic susceptibility or resistance are in development by a variety of different biotech companies. It will be critical for ASPs to partner with their clinical laboratory as new assays, especially those providing more comprehensive genotypic antimicrobial resistance information, become available in the future.

LRTI is also an active area of diagnostic device development. Clinical trials of a FilmArray (Biofire Diagnostics, Salt Lake City, UT, USA) multiplex LRTI panel that includes semiquantitative assessment of multiple bacterial targets, viral pathogens, and several resistance genes are underway.[55] In addition, laboratory-developed unbiased metagenomic approaches using massively parallel next-generation sequencing (NGS) are being developed to detect all possible pathogens. Interpreting the results of these assays in the setting of a patient with LRTI is anticipated to be complex. Neither of these approaches can separate organisms colonizing the respiratory tract or oropharynx from those causing invasive lower tract disease; whether semiquantitation of molecular results will be useful in this regard is not known. Given these issues, advanced diagnostics for LRTI will be prime candidates for ASP oversight.

In the future, it is also anticipated that measures of host immune responses via gene expression profiling will be used to help diagnose infectious diseases. The human immune responses to infection as compared with noninfectious inflammatory conditions are different and viral versus bacterial responses are also unique. Host-based transcriptomics have mainly been evaluated in the setting of sepsis and respiratory tract infection.[56,57] Preliminary assessments, at least for immune competent patients, seem promising and one can easily envision multiplex PCR panels or NGS reports that integrate pathogen detection and with measures of the host response.

In the clinical microbiology laboratory, molecular and proteomic revolution has created a need for more implementation science and outcome studies to help determine best use of new tests. Three ongoing studies, sponsored at least in part by the Antibiotic Leadership Group,[58] have been designed to specifically assess use of PCT or host-response signatures in patients presenting with signs of respiratory tract infection as well as to determine the potential clinical impact of rapid phenotypic susceptibility testing in patients with Gram-negative bacteremia.[59] Although pre-/postintervention studies can be informative, future research should ideally include prospective assessments of antimicrobial utilization, clinical outcomes, and health care costs associated with new diagnostic strategies.

SUMMARY

Significant advances have been made in microbiology rapid diagnostics for BSIs, respiratory tract infections, and GI infections, with newer technologies allowing for sensitive testing for multiple organisms at the same time. These technologies allow for earlier identification of infection and available evidence finds they reduce time to appropriate antimicrobial therapy and potentially improve clinical outcomes when coupled with ASP intervention. The strongest data exist for RDT for BSIs paired with ASP intervention, and additional outcomes studies are needed to assess the impact of RDT for respiratory tract infections and GI infections on antimicrobial use and clinical outcomes when paired with ASP intervention.

Rapid diagnostics have only begun to transform our ability to diagnose infectious diseases with more advanced technologies on the horizon. Looking forward, it is imperative that the appropriate implementation, clinical impact, and cost-effectiveness of new diagnostics be evaluated in relation to antimicrobial stewardship efforts as stewardship expands across the health care spectrum.

REFERENCES

1. Forrest GN, Roghmann MC, Toombs LS, et al. Peptide nucleic acid fluorescent in situ hybridization for hospital-acquired enterococcal bacteremia: delivering earlier effective antimicrobial therapy. Antimicrob Agents Chemother 2008; 52(10):3558–63.
2. Banerjee R, Teng CB, Cunningham SA, et al. Randomized trial of rapid multiplex polymerase chain reaction-based blood culture identification and susceptibility testing. Clin Infect Dis 2015;61(7):1071–80.
3. Barlam TF, Cosgrove SE, Abbo LM, et al. Implementing an antibiotic stewardship program: guidelines by the infectious diseases society of America and the society for healthcare epidemiology of America. Clin Infect Dis 2016; 62(10):e51–77.
4. Frye AM, Baker CA, Rustvold DL, et al. Clinical impact of a real-time PCR assay for rapid identification of staphylococcal bacteremia. J Clin Microbiol 2012;50(1): 127–33.
5. Cosgrove SE, Li DX, Tamma PD, et al. Use of PNA FISH for blood cultures growing Gram-positive cocci in chains without a concomitant antibiotic stewardship intervention does not improve time to appropriate antibiotic therapy. Diagn Microbiol Infect Dis 2016;86(1):86–92.
6. Holtzman C, Whitney D, Barlam T, et al. Assessment of impact of peptide nucleic acid fluorescence in situ hybridization for rapid identification of coagulase-negative staphylococci in the absence of antimicrobial stewardship intervention. J Clin Microbiol 2011;49(4):1581–2.
7. Pancholi P, Carroll KC, Buchan BW, et al. Multicenter evaluation of the accelerate phenotest BC Kit for rapid identification and phenotypic antimicrobial susceptibility testing using morphokinetic cellular analysis. J Clin Microbiol 2018. https://doi.org/10.1128/JCM.01329-17.
8. Forrest GN, Mehta S, Weekes E, et al. Impact of rapid in situ hybridization testing on coagulase-negative staphylococci positive blood cultures. J Antimicrob Chemother 2006;58(1):154–8.
9. Bauer KA, West JE, Balada-Llasat JM, et al. An antimicrobial stewardship program's impact with rapid polymerase chain reaction methicillin-resistant Staphylococcus aureus/S. aureus blood culture test in patients with S. aureus bacteremia. Clin Infect Dis 2010;51(9):1074–80.

10. Perez KK, Olsen RJ, Musick WL, et al. Integrating rapid pathogen identification and antimicrobial stewardship significantly decreases hospital costs. Arch Pathol Lab Med 2013;137(9):1247–54.

11. Huang AM, Newton D, Kunapuli A, et al. Impact of rapid organism identification via matrix-assisted laser desorption/ionization time-of-flight combined with antimicrobial stewardship team intervention in adult patients with bacteremia and candidemia. Clin Infect Dis 2013;57(9):1237–45.

12. Walker T, Dumadag S, Lee CJ, et al. Clinical impact of laboratory implementation of verigene BC-GN microarray-based assay for detection of gram-negative bacteria in positive blood cultures. J Clin Microbiol 2016;54(7):1789–96.

13. MacVane SH, Hurst JM, Boger MS, et al. Impact of a rapid multiplex polymerase chain reaction blood culture identification technology on outcomes in patients with vancomycin-resistant Enterococcal bacteremia. Infect Dis (Lond) 2016; 48(10):732–7.

14. Cairns KA, Doyle JS, Trevillyan JM, et al. The impact of a multidisciplinary antimicrobial stewardship team on the timeliness of antimicrobial therapy in patients with positive blood cultures: a randomized controlled trial. J Antimicrob Chemother 2016;71(11):3276–83.

15. Timbrook TT, Morton JB, McConeghy KW, et al. The effect of molecular rapid diagnostic testing on clinical outcomes in bloodstream infections: a systematic review and meta-analysis. Clin Infect Dis 2017;64(1):15–23.

16. McElvania TeKippe E. The added cost of rapid diagnostic testing and active antimicrobial stewardship: is it worth it? J Clin Microbiol 2017;55(1):20–3.

17. Patel TS, Kaakeh R, Nagel JL, et al. Cost analysis of implementing matrix-assisted laser desorption ionization-time of flight mass spectrometry plus real-time antimicrobial stewardship intervention for bloodstream infections. J Clin Microbiol 2017;55(1):60–7.

18. Brown J, Paladino JA. Impact of rapid methicillin-resistant Staphylococcus aureus polymerase chain reaction testing on mortality and cost effectiveness in hospitalized patients with bacteraemia: a decision model. Pharmacoeconomics 2010;28(7):567–75.

19. Wilson NAG, Tibbetts RJ, Samuel LP, et al. T2 magnetic resonance assay improves timely management of Candidemia. J Antimicrob Steward 2017; 1(1):12–8.

20. Garey KW, Rege M, Pai MP, et al. Time to initiation of fluconazole therapy impacts mortality in patients with candidemia: a multi-institutional study. Clin Infect Dis 2006;43(1):25–31.

21. Patel GP, Simon D, Scheetz M, et al. The effect of time to antifungal therapy on mortality in Candidemia associated septic shock. Am J Ther 2009;16(6):508–11.

22. Forrest GN, Mankes K, Jabra-Rizk MA, et al. Peptide nucleic acid fluorescence in situ hybridization-based identification of Candida albicans and its impact on mortality and antifungal therapy costs. J Clin Microbiol 2006;44(9):3381–3.

23. Heil EL, Daniels LM, Long DM, et al. Impact of a rapid peptide nucleic acid fluorescence in situ hybridization assay on treatment of Candida infections. Am J Health Syst Pharm 2012;69(21):1910–4.

24. Bilir SP, Ferrufino CP, Pfaller MA, et al. The economic impact of rapid Candida species identification by T2Candida among high-risk patients. Future Microbiol 2015;10(7):1133–44.

25. Walker B, Powers-Fletcher MV, Schmidt RL, et al. Cost-effectiveness analysis of multiplex PCR with magnetic resonance detection versus empiric or blood

culture-directed therapy for management of suspected Candidemia. J Clin Microbiol 2016;54(3):718–26.

26. Brendish NJ, Malachira AK, Armstrong L, et al. Routine molecular point-of-care testing for respiratory viruses in adults presenting to hospital with acute respiratory illness (ResPOC): a pragmatic, open-label, randomised controlled trial. Lancet Respir Med 2017;5(5):401–11.

27. Rappo U, Schuetz AN, Jenkins SG, et al. Impact of early detection of respiratory viruses by multiplex PCR assay on clinical outcomes in adult patients. J Clin Microbiol 2016;54(8):2096–103.

28. Green DA, Hitoaliaj L, Kotansky B, et al. Clinical utility of on-demand multiplex respiratory pathogen testing among adult outpatients. J Clin Microbiol 2016; 54(12):2950–5.

29. Semret M, Schiller I, Jardin BA, et al. Multiplex respiratory virus testing for antimicrobial stewardship: a prospective assessment of antimicrobial use and clinical outcomes among hospitalized adults. J Infect Dis 2017;216(8): 936–44.

30. Hersh AL, Shapiro DJ, Pavia AT, et al. Antibiotic prescribing in ambulatory pediatrics in the United States. Pediatrics 2011;128(6):1053–61.

31. Schuetz P, Wirz Y, Sager R, et al. Effect of procalcitonin-guided antibiotic treatment on mortality in acute respiratory infections: a patient level meta-analysis. Lancet Infect Dis 2018;18(1):95–107.

32. Timbrook T, Maxam M, Bosso J. Antibiotic discontinuation rates associated with positive respiratory viral panel and low procalcitonin results in proven or suspected respiratory infections. Infect Dis Ther 2015;4(3):297–306.

33. Parente DM, Cunha CB, Mylonakis E, et al. The Clinical utility of methicillin resistant Staphylococcus aureus (MRSA) nasal screening to rule out MRSA pneumonia: a diagnostic meta-analysis with antimicrobial stewardship implications. Clin Infect Dis 2018. https://doi.org/10.1093/cid/ciy024.

34. Smith MN, Erdman MJ, Ferreira JA, et al. Clinical utility of methicillin-resistant Staphylococcus aureus nasal polymerase chain reaction assay in critically ill patients with nosocomial pneumonia. J Crit Care 2017;38:168–71.

35. Willis C, Allen B, Tucker C, et al. Impact of a pharmacist-driven methicillin-resistant Staphylococcus aureus surveillance protocol. Am J Health Syst Pharm 2017; 74(21):1765–73.

36. Koo HL, Van JN, Zhao M, et al. Real-time polymerase chain reaction detection of asymptomatic Clostridium difficile colonization and rising C. difficile-associated disease rates. Infect Control Hosp Epidemiol 2014;35(6): 667–73.

37. Truong CY, Gombar S, Wilson R, et al. Real-time electronic tracking of diarrheal episodes and laxative therapy enables verification of clostridium difficile clinical testing criteria and reduction of clostridium difficile infection rates. J Clin Microbiol 2017;55(5):1276–84.

38. Buckel WR, Avdic E, Carroll KC, et al. Gut check: Clostridium difficile testing and treatment in the molecular testing era. Infect Control Hosp Epidemiol 2015;36(2): 217–21.

39. Ahmad SM, Blanco N, Dewart CM, et al. Laxative use in the setting of positive testing for Clostridium difficile infection. Infect Control Hosp Epidemiol 2017; 38(12):1513–5.

40. Brumley PE, Malani AN, Kabara JJ, et al. Effect of an antimicrobial stewardship bundle for patients with Clostridium difficile infection. J Antimicrob Chemother 2016;71(3):836–40.

41. Jury LA, Tomas M, Kundrapu S, et al. A Clostridium difficile infection (CDI) stewardship initiative improves adherence to practice guidelines for management of CDI. Infect Control Hosp Epidemiol 2013;34(11):1222–4.

42. Welch HK, Nagel JL, Patel TS, et al. Effect of an antimicrobial stewardship intervention on outcomes for patients with Clostridium difficile infection. Am J Infect Control 2016;44(12):1539–43.

43. Polen CB, Judd WR, Ratliff PD, et al. Impact of real-time notification of Clostridium difficile test results and early initiation of effective antimicrobial therapy. Am J Infect Control 2018. https://doi.org/10.1016/j.ajic.2017.11.010.

44. Beal SG, Tremblay EE, Toffel S, et al. A gastrointestinal PCR panel improves clinical management and lowers health care costs. J Clin Microbiol 2018;56(1) [pii: e01457-17].

45. Raux BR, Aldhaeefi M, Steed LL, et al. Utilization of filmarray gastrointestinal panel (GIP) results on altering empiric antibiotic (ABX) use in patients with acute diarrhea. Open Forum Infect Dis 2017;4(suppl_1):S604.

46. ISRCTNregistry. Point-of-care testing for gastrointestinal pathogens. 2018. Available at: www.isrctn.com/ISRCTN88918395. Accessed February 9, 2018.

47. Goldenberg SD, Bacelar M, Brazier P, et al. A cost benefit analysis of the Luminex xTAG gastrointestinal pathogen panel for detection of infectious gastroenteritis in hospitalised patients. J Infect 2015;70(5):504–11.

48. Donner LM, Campbell WS, Lyden E, et al. Assessment of rapid-blood-culture-identification result interpretation and antibiotic prescribing practices. J Clin Microbiol 2017;55(5):1496–507.

49. Messacar K, Hurst AL, Child J, et al. Clinical impact and provider acceptability of real-time antimicrobial stewardship decision support for rapid diagnostics in children with positive blood culture results. J Pediatric Infect Dis Soc 2017;6(3):267–74.

50. Messacar K, Parker SK, Todd JK, et al. Implementation of rapid molecular infectious disease diagnostics: the role of diagnostic and antimicrobial stewardship. J Clin Microbiol 2017;55(3):715–23.

51. Wenzler E, Timbrook T, Wong J, et al. Implementation and optimization of molecular rapid diagnostics in bloodstream infections: a clinical review. Am J Health Syst Pharm, in press.

52. Dellinger RP, Levy MM, Rhodes A, et al. Surviving sepsis campaign: international guidelines for management of severe sepsis and septic shock: 2012. Crit Care Med 2013;41(2):580–637.

53. Kumar A, Ellis P, Arabi Y, et al. Initiation of inappropriate antimicrobial therapy results in a fivefold reduction of survival in human septic shock. Chest 2009;136(5):1237–48.

54. T2Biosystems. T2Bacteria panel. 2018. Available at: www.t2biosystems.com/t2sepsis-solution/t2bacteria-panel/. Accessed February 9, 2018.

55. ClinicalTrials.gov. Clinical Evaluation of FilmArray LRTI Panel. 2018. Available at: clinicaltrials.gov/ct2/show/NCT02929680. Accessed February 9, 2018.

56. Ginsburg GS, Woods CW. The host response to infection: advancing a novel diagnostic paradigm. Crit Care 2012;16(6):168.

57. Holcomb ZE, Tsalik EL, Woods CW, et al. Host-based peripheral blood gene expression analysis for diagnosis of infectious diseases. J Clin Microbiol 2017;55(2):360–8.

58. Tsalik EL, Petzold E, Kreiswirth BN, et al. Advancing diagnostics to address antibacterial resistance: the diagnostics and devices committee of the antibacterial resistance leadership group. Clin Infect Dis 2017;64(suppl_1):S41–7.

59. Antibacterial Resistance Leadership Group. Studies In Progress. 2017. Available at: www.arlg.org/studies-in-progress. Accessed February 9, 2018.

Antimicrobial Stewardship in Community Hospitals

Whitney R. Buckel, PharmD[a],*, John J. Veillette, PharmD[b], Todd J. Vento, MD, MPH[c], Edward Stenehjem, MD, MSc[d]

KEYWORDS

- Antibiotic stewardship • Antimicrobial stewardship • Community hospitals
- Critical access hospitals • Small hospitals • Rural hospitals
- Antibiotic stewardship core elements

KEY POINTS

- Antibiotic stewardship programs are needed in all health care facilities, regardless of size and location.
- Antibiotic stewardship team leaders require dedicated administrative support to actively engage local prescribers.
- Antibiotic stewardship metrics that are actionable should be tracked and reported.
- Available resources and leadership priorities should be considered when selecting antibiotic stewardship goals and projects.

INTRODUCTION

In an era of health care when pressures to improve safety and quality and reduce waste are increasing, antimicrobial stewardship programs (ASPs) provide value by optimizing antimicrobial prescribing, improving clinical outcomes, and decreasing cost. In hospitals, one-third of antimicrobial prescribing is thought to be either unnecessary or inappropriate.[1] Formal ASPs can successfully respond to these health care pressures and reduce inappropriate antimicrobial use.

Disclosures: W.R. Buckel has received honoraria from Merck Co. for serving as a planning committee member for the Society for Healthcare Epidemiology of America's Antibiotic Stewardship Research Workshop. E. Stenehjem has received grant funding from The Joint Commission, Pfizer's Independent Grants for Learning and Change, Allergan, and AHRQ. T.J. Vento and J.J. Veillette have nothing to disclose.

[a] Intermountain Healthcare Pharmacy Services, 4292 South Riverboat Road, Suite 100, Taylorsville, UT 84123, USA; [b] Division of Infectious Diseases and Epidemiology, Intermountain Infectious Diseases TeleHealth Service, 5121 South Cottonwood Drive, Murray, UT 84107, USA; [c] Intermountain Infectious Diseases TeleHealth Service, 5121 South Cottonwood Drive, Murray, UT 84107, USA; [d] Intermountain Healthcare and TeleHealth Service, 5121 South Cottonwood Drive, Murray, UT 84107, USA
* Corresponding author.
E-mail address: whitney.buckel@imail.org

Since 1997, the Infectious Diseases Society of America (IDSA) and Society for Healthcare Epidemiology of America (SHEA) have recommended that every hospital regardless of size have an ASP.[2] More recently, the regulatory landscape has changed significantly to support the expansion of antimicrobial stewardship. In 2013, Accreditation Canada expanded the list of Required Organizational Practices to include development and implementation of a program to optimize antimicrobial use and provide good stewardship. In 2014 and 2015, respectively, the Canadian and US governments released national action plans to address antimicrobial resistance.[3,4] In the United States, this led The Joint Commission to implement a new medication management standard on January 1, 2017, requiring active ASPs at all accredited hospitals.[5] Critical access hospitals will need to comply with the Centers for Disease Control and Prevention (CDC) Core Elements[6] of Antibiotic Stewardship by 2021 to receive flexibility (flex) grant funding from the Federal Office of Rural Health Policy via the Medicare Beneficiary Quality Improvement Project (MBQIP).[7] The Centers for Medicaid and Medicare Services (CMS) drafted a proposal to require ASPs as a condition of participation.[8] Individual states, to include California and Missouri, have their own stewardship requirements.[1] Importantly, all guidelines, regulatory recommendations, and accreditation standards require the implementation of an ASP regardless of hospital size, academic affiliation, or location.

The impact of ASPs has largely been studied in academic medical centers.[9] However, academic medical centers account for only 400 of the more than 4800 nonfederal, acute care hospitals in the United States.[10,11] The remaining 4400 are community hospitals, and most of these are small community hospitals with fewer than 200 beds. These smaller facilities represent 72% of US nonfederal hospitals and are least likely to have an ASP that meets all of the CDC's Core Elements.[12,13] Compared with academic medical centers, community hospitals face unique challenges that require different and creative approaches to antimicrobial stewardship. The purpose of this article is to compare and contrast these challenges and to propose strategies for community hospitals to meet the CDC Core Elements.

Agreeing on one definition of a community hospital is challenging.[14] For the purposes of this review, community hospitals are defined as nonfederal, short-term general hospitals that are not academic medical centers or major teaching hospitals. Community hospitals represent a diverse group ranging from a 20-bed, rural, critical access hospital, to a 600-bed, urban, multispecialty hospital. Because of the significant heterogeneity among community hospitals, this review article at times separates the discussion of stewardship approaches based on the hospital categories defined in **Table 1**. Even within these categories, there can be significant variability due to hospitals being private or public, for-profit or nonprofit, or part of a network or system. There may be differences between hospitals in terms of rounding structures, presence of students and/or residents, research activities, access to journal articles, patient acuity level, likelihood to transfer patients, capabilities of on-site microbiology laboratories, and presence of intensive care units, on-site subspecialists, and transplant services. It is important to keep this heterogeneity in mind as we compare and contrast stewardship in community and academic settings. The recommendations in this article are largely based on the authors' collective experience working with community hospitals in the mountain west region.

LEADERSHIP COMMITMENT
Similarities

Regardless of hospital size, leadership support is critical to the development and sustainability of an ASP. Hospital leadership must understand the importance of the ASP

Table 1
Example characteristics of community hospitals based on bed size and location

	Small (<200 beds)[b]	Medium/Large (≥200 beds)[b]
Urban[a] (county population 50,000 or greater)	Hospital SU is an 89-bed facility located in a city with a population of approximately 28,000 situated only 12 miles from a large tertiary hospital in a city of more than 100,000 people. The pharmacy is open 24 hours a day, 7 days a week. The hospital offers women and newborn, surgical, and cancer services. There is 1 small ICU. There is no on-site ID physician, although the ID physician at the nearby hospital will provide phone consultation and occasional on-site consultation.	Hospital LU is a 395-bed facility located in a city with a population of more than 100,000 people. The pharmacy is open 24 hours a day, 7 days a week, with pharmacy specialist services, including an ID pharmacist. It is a level II Trauma Center. The hospital offers many subspecialty services, including advanced cardiovascular care. There are 2 ICUs. The hospital trains family medicine residents and has a pharmacy residency program. There is 1 on-site ID physician.
Rural[a] (county population <50,000)	Hospital RS is an 18-bed critical access hospital in a city of approximately 3000 people. It is located almost 100 miles from the closest tertiary hospital. The pharmacy is open Monday through Friday business hours, operated by 1 pharmacist. The hospital primarily offers emergency services and is mostly staffed by family practice physicians. There is no on-site ID physician.	Hospital MR is a 230-bed facility located 80 miles outside a large urban city and 23 miles away from the nearest hospital. It serves 9 counties and has 29 employed physicians, including a recently hired ID physician. The pharmacy is open 7 days a week, but no overnight coverage.

Abbreviations: ICU, intensive care unit; ID, infectious diseases.

[a] There are challenges in defining rural from a health care perspective. For the purpose of this review, we consider rural as any nonmetropolitan county (counties with a population of <50,000).[66]

[b] There is no clear cutoff between small and medium/large facilities; however, for the purpose of this article we use a cutoff of 200 beds.[67]

in improving patient outcomes, mitigating antimicrobial resistance, and meeting regulatory requirements.[15,16] Accordingly, leadership needs to dedicate time and resources to antimicrobial stewardship, and they should be informed about the projects, activities, and goals of the stewardship team. Hospital leadership also can provide motivation and accountability for team members, support the ASP when problems or resource issues arise, and increase the awareness of stewardship within the institution. Stewardship programs are more likely to be successful if their projects are aligned with organization and leadership goals.

Differences

Due to limited resources, the leadership structure may vary significantly in community hospitals when compared with academic medical centers. Often, community hospitals have fewer hospital administrators, but they might be more involved with day-to-day hospital activities. This can be helpful in demonstrating how an ASP would improve patient care. In small community hospitals, the needs of an ASP might not require the addition of a full-time staff member, as opposed to academic medical centers that often require multiple pharmacists and/or physicians to conduct ASP activities. However, hospital leadership will need to designate protected stewardship time for existing staff, which can pose additional challenges for small facilities.

Strategies

In all settings, a letter of support from leadership is a great start; however, it is typically not enough to fully support an ASP. Engaging hospital leadership to be involved in setting goals and expectations and securing ASP resources is critical. When possible, we recommend including administrative leaders as members of the ASP and sharing the impact of ASP interventions to develop and maintain a successful relationship. See the sections that follow on accountability, drug expertise, and key support for more information on potential financial requests. Grant funding also can be used to help support ASP pilot projects and to help evaluate the potential benefit of securing additional resources.[17]

ACCOUNTABILITY AND DRUG EXPERTISE
Similarities

Every hospital needs local, on-site, antimicrobial stewardship champions for accountability and drug expertise purposes.[6] Ideally, the designated lead(s) should be respected by their peers, willing to participate in the program, and have protected time for their antimicrobial stewardship responsibilities. National guidelines recommend infectious diseases (ID)-trained clinicians provide this leadership.[18] ASPs are frequently co-led by a physician and pharmacist, both with ID postgraduate training.[19,20]

Differences

In academic medical centers and large community hospitals, ID-trained physicians and pharmacists are often employed or contracted by the hospital and should be included as leaders of the ASP. However, this ASP structure is not realistic in small community hospitals where ID-trained physicians and pharmacists are rare. In a 2010 survey of hospitals with mostly fewer than 300 beds, only 58.8% had access to an on-site ID physician.[21] In Colorado, none of their rural hospitals had access to ID physicians.[22] Similarly, in Utah, only 1 of Intermountain Healthcare's 15 small community hospitals had access to on-site ID consultation in 2014. In facilities without ID-trained physicians, alternative stewardship leaders will need to be sought and may require additional training and education.

Pharmacy staffing structures are often different at community hospitals. As hospital size decreases, pharmacists are less likely to be residency trained or specialized in a particular area.[23] The smallest sites may have only 1 pharmacist, let alone 1 ID pharmacist. Community hospital pharmacies might contract externally for their order entry needs. Even having a single ID pharmacist presents some challenges with covering paid time off compared with facilities with multiple ID pharmacists.

Strategies

ASPs at community hospitals have taken many forms in terms of accountability and drug expertise leadership. ASPs have been led by an ID physician alone,[24] an ID pharmacist alone,[25] an ID physician and ID pharmacist team,[17,26,27] an ID physician with non-ID clinical pharmacist,[28–31] an ID provider located off-site that provided support to local physicians and pharmacists,[32–34] and without any support from ID-trained providers.[35,36] The final structure of a community hospital's ASP will require efficient use of available resources.

Community hospitals in close proximity to urban settings should consider recruiting nearby ID-trained physicians to participate in their ASP.[24] The time commitment will vary based on the hospital size, pharmacist resources, availability of local physician champions, and expected responsibilities, and may range from 1 to 10, or even more, hours per week.[29,32,37] Appropriate compensation for their time will be required for a sustainable program. An international survey recommended 0.1 physician full-time equivalent (FTE) for every 100 beds.[38]

Often, ID-trained physicians will not be available to participate in the ASP. In this case, identifying and engaging local physicians is another solution. These physicians are often internal medicine or family medicine providers, but if at an orthopedic specialty hospital, perhaps an orthopedic surgeon would maximize buy-in from fellow surgeons. Hospitalists are well-positioned to lead stewardship efforts and provide accountability and drug expertise.[39,40] Hospital leadership should facilitate additional training for local ASP leaders, especially those who lack formal ID training. Possibilities include online programs provided by SHEA, IDSA, Stanford, Society of Infectious Diseases Pharmacist, Making a Difference in Infectious Diseases, and others or shadowing ASP personnel at other hospitals. Telehealth services are another option to provide ID expertise and mentorship to local ASP leaders. Telehealth solutions can take the form of telephone consultations,[32] Extension for Community Healthcare Outcomes (ECHO) education models,[41] or a consultation provided within a health system with the same electronic medical record.[34]

Pharmacists also can provide accountability and drug expertise in community hospitals. Large community hospitals should support a dedicated ASP pharmacist with ID training. An international survey suggested at least 1 pharmacist FTE for every 300 beds dedicated to stewardship.[38] Dedicated ASP pharmacists should ideally have the responsibilities written into their contract(s) and/or job description(s) regardless of hospital size. Examples of community hospitals that have successfully implemented ASPs without an ID-trained pharmacist did so with either a dedicated antimicrobial stewardship shift[29,37] or by incorporating stewardship activities into clinical pharmacists' daily responsibilities.[17,28,42] Assigning antimicrobial stewardship activities to pharmacists with other responsibilities may lead to a lower percentage of patients reviewed due to competing priorities[27] and can be partially counteracted by providing protected time.[42] In the authors' experience, consistency is key to the success of stewardship interventions and rotating stewardship responsibilities through multiple shifts or pharmacists is often problematic. Ideally, pharmacists that provide drug expertise for the ASP should have additional training, such as those listed previously for physicians. If additional training is not available, hospitals can seek remote coaching relationships with School of Pharmacy faculty,[17] local health departments or health authorities,[43] telelehealth,[34] or state-based collaboratives.[44]

Multidisciplinary team members

The work of ASP leaders is greatly enhanced by the support of a multidisciplinary team that may include infection preventionists, nurses, microbiologists, information technology (IT) personnel, data analysts, and antibiotic prescribers, such as nurse practitioners and physician assistants. In community hospitals, particularly those that are small, this team may not include all of the key support personnel recommended in national guidelines and CDC's Core Elements. Identifying staff that are interested in supporting stewardship is more important than the titles they hold. Using all available resources in small hospitals may take creativity and be unique to individual hospitals. Examples of engaging interested staff include the following:

- Pharmacy technicians often gather medication histories and can be useful to include in an antibiotic allergy screening initiative.[35]
- Trainees (eg, students and residents) can be involved in the daily tasks of antibiotic stewardship.[17,29,32,45,46]
- In optimizing surgical prophylaxis, consider engaging the infection preventionist.[47]
- At one site, the chief medical officer was actively engaged in reviewing patients on targeted antimicrobials.[32]

ACTION
Similarities

Currently, prospective audit with intervention and feedback (PAWIF) and restriction with prior authorization are the 2 main pillars of antimicrobial stewardship in the inpatient setting, regardless of hospital size or location.[18] An antibiotic time-out (ATO) is an example of another action that has been shown to improve antibiotic prescribing.[46] Additional interventions that are used in both academic medical centers and community hospitals can be categorized as drug-specific, syndrome-specific, or process-specific (**Table 2**). All interventions, including diagnostic and treatment guidelines, are best when modified to fit the local setting.

Differences

PAWIF, restrictions, and ATO require the stewardship team to be alerted when antibiotics are used or ordered. In smaller hospitals, the stewardship team may be able to review every patient receiving antibiotics, but also may have less time and resources to do so. In larger community hospitals, reviewing all patients receiving antibiotics is time consuming and labor intensive. In either case, IT solutions within an electronic health record or third-party computer decision support software can improve efficiency.[48–50] However, these electronic tools and IT support may not be available in all community hospitals. In academic medical centers, ID fellows often manage antibiotic restrictions. In community hospitals, where fellows are typically absent, antibiotic restriction policies need to be adapted to local staffing and resources.

Microbiology laboratory–based stewardship initiatives are often challenging in community hospitals as many laboratories are off-site or contracted to large, centralized laboratories. These hospitals often do not have a relationship with the microbiology laboratory director, have longer turnaround times, lack access to rapid diagnostic tests like matric-assisted laser desorption ionization time of flight, and suffer from limited communication with microbiology laboratory technicians.

Strategies

In our experience, stewardship strategies can be tailored to any setting, whether urban or rural, small or large. A simple ATO may be the easiest to implement, as it is a simple reminder to the prescriber to reevaluate the antibiotic course and can be initiated by anyone on the health care team.[40] An advanced version of the ATO is PAWIF, in which specific recommendations are made by the ASP team based on appropriateness guidelines or a checklist (**Fig. 1** shows a checklist developed at Intermountain Healthcare). Because PAWIF can be time intensive, resource-constrained settings can

Table 2
Actionable, intervention-based metrics to consider by topic

Topic	Possible Metrics	Potential Action
Drug-specific Examples: • Meropenem MUE • Clindamycin MUE • All broad-spectrum	• Number of doses per month • DOT or DDD per 1000 patient days (present) • Acquisition cost • % appropriate (criteria-based, route-based, dosing/renal adjustment-based) • Antibiotic-related ADRs (such as AKI or high vancomycin troughs)	• Education on appropriateness • Restriction • Prospective audit and feedback • STOP and review at order entry
Disease-specific Examples: • CAP • UTI/ASB • Bloodstream infections	• % guideline adherent treatment • % appropriate route • Length of therapy • Rate of *Clostridium difficile*[a] • Length of stay (ICU/hospital) • Readmissions[a] • Mortality[a]	• Guideline development • Guideline promotion, education, and integration into CPOE • Prospective audit and feedback (eg, daily review of positive blood cultures, urine cultures and/or S pneumoniae urinary antigen testing)
Process-specific Examples: • Rapid diagnostics • Allergy assessment • ED culture follow-up	• Time to appropriate antibiotics • % adherence to policies • % allergies with a documented reaction • No. patients with cultures reviewed within __ time • No. patients in whom antibiotic therapy was changed based on culture follow-up • No. (%) of patients who received empiric therapy that covered the organism that grew	• Standard operating procedures • Changes in the electronic health record • Guideline development • Education • Micro laboratory calls to pharmacy with rapid diagnostic results

Abbreviations: ADR, adverse drug reaction; AKI, acute kidney injury; ASB, asymptomatic bacteriuria; CAP, community-acquired pneumonia; CPOE, computerized prescriber order entry; DDD, defined daily doses; DOT, days of therapy; ED, emergency department; ICU, intensive care unit; MUE, medication use evaluation; UTI, urinary tract infection.
[a] May be challenging for small facilities to demonstrate meaningful change.

consider limiting the audits to 3 times a week,[37,51] twice a week,[31] or even once weekly with an ID physician.[24,32] PAWIF can be initially started on select units, such as internal medicine floors or intensive care units.[28,31] PAWIF also can be triggered by the use of specific drugs or drug classes (eg, fluoroquinolones) or certain microbiology results (eg, positive blood cultures). Screening tools for these triggers can be challenging to obtain, as described previously, but can be provided by a third-party application,[37,49] by building reports into existing programs,[30] or by collaborating with the microbiology laboratory.[30,42]

Antibiotic restrictions may be more impactful in small community hospitals,[52] but the effectiveness of restrictions compared with PAWIF has not been formally assessed in this setting and may have unintended consequences, such as delayed antibiotic therapy.[53,54] In the absence of ID fellows approving restricted antibiotics, community

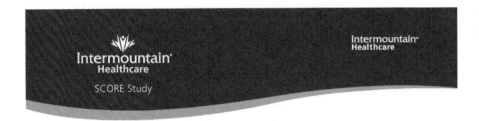

▶ **Antimicrobial Stewardship Checklist — *High***

Print a list of patients on antibiotics for your coverage area. Review each prescribed antibiotic for the following.

Antibiotic Indication

☐ Review for *Antimicrobial Indication*[a] and concordance with the *Antimicrobial Prescribing Procedures*.

Antibiotic Restrictions

☐ Determine if antimicrobial is a *Restricted Antimicrobial* and follow up pending approvals.

Microbiology

☐ Review **microbiology** to evaluate for *Bug-Drug Mismatch*.
☐ **For patients with positive clinical cultures only!** Review all patients on vancomycin, imipenem, meropenem, ertapenem, piperacillin/tazobactam, cefepime, aminoglycosides, ceftriaxone, levofloxacin, and/or ciprofloxacin per the *De-escalation* protocol.
☐ Determine if there is duplicate or missing treatment for *Anaerobes*.
☐ Determine if the syndrome present meets criteria for *When to Consult Infectious Diseases*.

Dose, Route, and Administration

☐ Review antimicrobial **dose and frequency** based on indication, patient weight, and patient renal function; refer to *Antimicrobial Dosing Guidelines* for assistance.
☐ Review antimicrobial **route** to determine if *IV to PO conversion* should be recommended.
☐ Review antimicrobial for **duration**.

Fig. 1. Sample antibiotic stewardship checklist. [a] More detail about these procedures is available on the SCORE Study page of intermountain.net. Search for "SCORE Study" or navigate to quality and patient safety. (© 2014 Intermountain Healthcare. Used with permission.)

hospitals can train front-line pharmacists to enforce restrictions, use a smaller list of restricted drugs, and have a more liberal restriction policy on nights and weekends.[33] If possible, the electronic medical record can support an approval process.[55] In our experience, restriction by centralized ID pharmacists and physicians was more effective at reducing broad-spectrum antibiotic use than local restriction; however, on-site restriction can be effective at individual sites, especially when supported by the local antibiogram.[56]

Focusing on syndrome-specific interventions targeting urinary tract infections, pneumonia, skin and soft tissue infections, and surgical prophylaxis is an alternative strategy that can be used in community hospitals. Institution-specific guidelines can be adapted from national guidelines created by organizations such as IDSA, SHEA, the CDC, and the American Thoracic Society. Institution-specific guidelines should be tailored to local antibiograms, distributed to the medical staff, and posted on the hospital intranet. Simple and well-studied initiatives, such as duration of therapy for community-acquired pneumonia[27,44] or guideline recommendations for surgical prophylaxis,[47] might be easier than interventions involving diagnosis if the ASP physician champion is not involved on a daily basis. Resources developed by other institutions can be used as a template for local development, especially for developing criteria for use for specific drugs.

With regard to implementation of policies and procedures, consider initially limiting the scope of those that are controversial and expanding after successful implementation may be an ideal approach.[42] Even if the initial acceptance rate is low, persistence is often successful in the long run.[24]

TRACKING: MONITORING ANTIBIOTIC PRESCRIBING, USE, AND RESISTANCE
Similarities

Regardless of size and academic affiliation, all ASPs need to track and measure aspects of antibiotic prescribing and the effectiveness of ASP interventions. This helps to identify inappropriate prescribing and demonstrate the effectiveness (or ineffectiveness) of a stewardship intervention. Measures used by ASPs include process, antibiotic consumption, and clinical outcome measures. A full discussion of ASP measures is out of the scope of this review, but many high-quality reviews are available.[57–60] Antibiotic consumption measures are most commonly used, but may not equate to appropriateness or clinical outcomes. Antibiotic prescribing appropriateness is also widely used but has varying definitions and can be laborious to determine.

Differences

The biggest difference among academic medical centers and community hospitals with regard to tracking is availability of antibiotic consumption data. Many community hospitals do not have access to IT support to assist with obtaining data for tracking and monitoring outcomes. Most of these facilities are left to obtain data manually or use nonvalidated sources for data extraction. In small hospitals, sample sizes are small and, regardless of the metric, significant month-to-month variability will be present requiring longer data intervals (eg, quarterly data) to obtain accurate measures. Small sample sizes are particularly challenging for microbiology-related measures in small community hospitals, which can be problematic for creating a local antibiogram or tracking antimicrobial resistance over time.

Strategies

Hospitals and ASPs that lack access to electronic antibiotic consumption data will have to find alternative methods for data tracking. Often, defined daily doses can be manually calculated using pharmacy administrative or purchasing data.[17,31] In very small hospitals, manual calculation of days of therapy is possible with a daily review of all patients and careful tracking of antibiotics administered. Denominator data, patient days present or patient days, can be obtained from administrative data. Days of therapy per 1000 patient days present is the national standard[61] and allows for benchmarking against other hospitals. We have found such benchmarking to be useful in identifying outliers in antibiotic prescribing in our small community hospitals. Community hospitals can consider manual tracking of process measures using tally sheets or electronic spreadsheets.[17,29]

Despite difficulties in defining antibiotic appropriateness and acknowledging that the definition may vary from institution to institution, we have found tracking and reporting appropriateness to be an effective stewardship tool. Appropriateness of diagnosis and management may be evaluated in addition to treatment appropriateness. The CDC has created appropriateness guides for a number of syndromes that can be used.[62] National guidelines and/or ID experts at other institutions can be used to create local guidelines for specific syndromes or the use of specific antimicrobials. The antibiotic stewardship team can then measure compliance with these guidelines after they have been implemented, using period point prevalence surveys. In assessing appropriateness, we recommend starting with high-volume conditions or specific antimicrobials first. Examples are provided in **Table 2**.

REPORTING
Similarities

All hospitals should consider establishing a formal reporting structure for their stewardship program. Antibiotic stewardship may report to a variety of upper-level committees or meetings, such as the Pharmacy and Therapeutics Committee, Quality and Patient Safety Committee, or Medical Executive Council, or a combination of these.[32,63] The best reporting structure for an institution's antibiotic stewardship program is not well defined and varies from institution to institution. In general, it is important to report pertinent data to the front-line staff providing patient care, administration, and quality and patient safety.

Differences

Reporting information to staff is very challenging, especially for nonemployed physicians who might not have clearly defined hospital-based reporting structures or institution-provided e-mail addresses. Smaller facilities might have fewer and less frequent meetings, further limiting communication of relevant ASP measures. Hospital committees might be combined at smaller facilities because leaders often wear multiple hats and it may be challenging to schedule meeting times.

Strategies

Some strategies to consider include online learning modules, placing informational posters in physician work areas, distributing pocket reference cards, developing antibiotic stewardship screensavers, and using existing newsletters. With regard to committee meetings, one approach is to request that antibiotic stewardship be a standing agenda item for an existing committee rather than hold a separate meeting, especially if key representatives are already in attendance.

EDUCATION
Similarities

Education is important, but is most effective when paired with an active intervention.[62] There are several examples of successful interventions that used education as a component of a multifaceted intervention.[27,64]

Differences

Nonacademic medical centers are less likely to provide routine formalized didactic lectures for their pharmacists and physicians. One-hour didactic lectures might also be unreasonable for clinicians with busy clinical practices, and these same clinicians also may be less responsive to e-mail given time constraints. Department meetings may be less frequent or absent in some facilities, which can make dissemination of information more challenging. Lack of on-site ID expertise may also limit opportunities to provide education.

Strategies

Anecdotally, a good starting place to educate providers is the local antibiogram and their prescribing patterns for certain disease states because it has led to changes in antibiotic prescribing. It is generally believed that in-person education is best, so although not always feasible, it might be worthwhile for remote ID mentors to travel for important education initiatives for added support and clarity. One strategy the authors have used is monthly 30-minute webinars. It is also important to remember that PAWIF, whether on a daily basis or a monthly basis,[65] is another form of effective education for all health care professionals. ID experts might be more persuasive when providing feedback and education regarding prescribing patterns for specific patient cases, and should be used if available.

WHERE TO BEGIN

Community hospitals have both limited resources and limited time under current financial pressures. In these settings, ASPs cannot tackle all stewardship problems in a sustainable manner. What might be considered low-hanging fruit at one facility can be challenging and controversial at another. However, gathering the right data or speaking to the right people can help identify an outlier, leading to a clear project choice. Some examples include broader than necessary empiric antibiotic therapy, delays in antibiotic therapy, inadequate antibiotic dosing or dose adjustments, missed opportunities to de-escalate, prolonged durations of therapy, or simply any area of extreme variation in prescribing. Improving processes such as allergy documentation or follow-up of finalized cultures also can provide value and improve care. **Table 3** provides additional guidance for antibiotic stewardship programs at various stages of development. Having a first, successful intervention is a win that not only demonstrates the worth of antimicrobial stewardship, but also builds confidence for future projects. There are also some practical, feasibility considerations:

- Consider the audience:
  - Align ASP goals and projects with leadership priorities.
  - Prioritize interventions that already have multidisciplinary buy-in.
  - Leverage respected health care workers and/or local experts.
- Consider the resources:
  - Do not tackle problems you do not have the resources to fix.
  - If you do not have a microbiology laboratory available, consider avoiding a microbiology-focused intervention.
  - If you do not have an ID physician or engaged physician champion, consider avoiding interventions related to diagnostics.
  - If you do not have an ID pharmacist, consider avoiding complicated medication use evaluations.

Table 3
Priority list of Interventions for Community Hospitals

Year	Goals	Interventions
<3 y	Small wins Demonstrate value	• Point prevalence surveys • Medication use evaluations • Positive blood and CSF culture review • Short list of restrictions • Short list of prospective audit and feedback • Other targeted initiatives: for example, d 3 of broad-spectrum antibiotics, HIV drug review, drug dosing initiatives
3–6 y	Sustainability New areas of impact	• Guideline development for common infections • Guideline adherence • Discharge antibiotic appropriateness
7+ y	Advanced interventions Validate new metrics "Community stewardship"	• Novel protocols and processes • More nuanced guidelines for rarer infections • Education of surrounding facilities

Abbreviations: CSF, cerebrospinal fluid; HIV, human immunodeficiency virus.

- Consider the impact:
  - Focus on what is common and has significant morbidity or mortality in your patient population.
  - Obtain data to help identify the areas for greatest improvement.
  - Start with tackling well-defined problems with clear solutions first.

FUTURE AREAS OF RESEARCH

More data are needed in many areas, including the following:

- The best structural and personnel components of a community hospital stewardship program
- Which structural components lead to successful interventions
- The role of central resources in networks and health systems
- The impact of telemedicine on antibiotic stewardship initiatives
- The role of existing health care worker relationships on implementing change

SUMMARY

The value and core framework of ASPs are similar between all hospital types; however, community hospitals that have fewer resources may have different priorities and require different strategies when defining ASP components and implementing interventions. By following the CDC Core Elements and using the strategies suggested in this article, readers should be able to design, develop, participate in, or improve ASPs within community hospitals. As previously described, ID pharmacists and physicians throughout North America are generally more than willing to "share advice, examples, and encouragement."[63] ASPs, via a systematic, coordinated approach with adequate accountability, can successfully respond to current health care pressures and reduce inappropriate antimicrobial use in hospitals of all sizes and locations.

REFERENCES

1. Antibiotic Use in the United States, 2017: Progress and Opportunities. 2017. Available at: https://www.cdc.gov/antibiotic-use/stewardship-report/hospital.html. Accessed February 1, 2018.

2. Shlaes DM, Gerding DN, John JF Jr, et al. Society for Healthcare Epidemiology of America and Infectious Diseases Society of America joint committee on the prevention of antimicrobial resistance: guidelines for the prevention of antimicrobial resistance in hospitals. Infect Control Hosp Epidemiol 1997;18:275–91.

3. Federal Action Plan on Antimicrobial Resistance and Use in Canada. 2015. Available at: http://healthycanadians.gc.ca/alt/pdf/publications/drugs-products-medicaments-produits/antibiotic-resistance-antibiotique/action-plan-daction-eng.pdf. Accessed February 1, 2018.

4. National Action Plan for Combating Antibiotic-Resistant Bacteria. 2015. Available at: https://www.cdc.gov/drugresistance/pdf/national_action_plan_for_combating_antibotic-resistant_bacteria.pdf. Accessed February 1, 2018.

5. Approved: New Antimicrobial Stewardship Standard. 2016. Available at: https://www.jointcommission.org/assets/1/6/New_Antimicrobial_Stewardship_Standard.pdf. Accessed February 1, 2018.

6. Implementation of Antibiotic Stewardship Core Elements at Small and Critical Access Hospitals. Available at: https://www.cdc.gov/antibiotic-use/healthcare/implementation/core-elements-small-critical.html. Accessed February 1, 2018.

7. MBQIP New Required Measure FY2018-2021. 2017. Available at: https://www.ruralcenter.org/file/antibiotics-stewardship-measures-mbqip-fiscal-years-2018-2021. Accessed February 1, 2018.

8. Medicare and Medicaid Programs; Hospital and Critical Access Hospital (CAH) Changes To Promote Innovation, Flexibility, and Improvement in Patient Care. 2016. Available at: https://www.federalregister.gov/documents/2016/06/16/2016-13925/medicare-and-medicaid-programs-hospital-and-critical-access-hospital-cah-changes-to-promote. Accessed February 1, 2018.

9. Trivedi KK, Kuper K. Hospital antimicrobial stewardship in the nonuniversity setting. Infect Dis Clin North Am 2014;28:281–9.

10. Fast Facts on U.S. Hospitals, 2018. 2018. Available at: https://www.aha.org/statistics/fast-facts-us-hospitals. Accessed February 1, 2018.

11. 50 things to know about the hospital industry | 2017. 2017. Available at: https://www.beckershospitalreview.com/hospital-management-administration/50-things-to-know-about-the-hospital-industry-2017.html. Accessed February 1, 2018.

12. National Center for Health Statistics, Health, United States. Health, United States, 2013: with special feature on prescription drugs. Hyattsville (MD): National Center for Health Statistics (US); 2014.

13. O'Leary EN, van Santen KL, Webb AK, et al. Uptake of antibiotic stewardship programs in US acute care hospitals: findings from the 2015 national healthcare safety network annual hospital survey. Clin Infect Dis 2017;65:1748–50.

14. The modern definition of a community hospital. 2015. Available at: https://www.beckershospitalreview.com/hospital-management-administration/the-modern-definition-of-a-community-hospital.html. Accessed February 1, 2018.

15. Spellberg B, Bartlett JG, Gilbert DN. How to pitch an antibiotic stewardship program to the hospital C-suite. Open Forum Infect Dis 2016;3:ofw210.

16. Nagel JL, Stevenson JG, Eiland EH 3rd, et al. Demonstrating the value of antimicrobial stewardship programs to hospital administrators. Clin Infect Dis 2014;59(Suppl 3):S146–53.

17. Lockwood AR, Bolton NS, Winton MD, et al. Formalization of an antimicrobial stewardship program in a small community hospital. Am J Health Syst Pharm 2017;74:S52–60.

18. Barlam TF, Cosgrove SE, Abbo LM, et al. Implementing an antibiotic stewardship program: guidelines by the Infectious Diseases Society of America and the Society for Healthcare Epidemiology of America. Clin Infect Dis 2016;62:e51–77.
19. Bessesen MT, Ma A, Clegg D, et al. Antimicrobial stewardship programs: comparison of a program with infectious diseases pharmacist support to a program with a geographic pharmacist staffing model. Hosp Pharm 2015;50:477–83.
20. Yu K, Rho J, Morcos M, et al. Evaluation of dedicated infectious diseases pharmacists on antimicrobial stewardship teams. Am J Health Syst Pharm 2014;71: 1019–28.
21. Septimus EJ, Owens RC Jr. Need and potential of antimicrobial stewardship in community hospitals. Clin Infect Dis 2011;53(Suppl 1):S8–14.
22. Reese SM, Gilmartin H, Rich KL, et al. Infection prevention needs assessment in Colorado hospitals: rural and urban settings. Am J Infect Control 2014;42: 597–601.
23. Pedersen CA, Schneider PJ, Scheckelhoff DJ. ASHP national survey of pharmacy practice in hospital settings: prescribing and transcribing-2016. Am J Health Syst Pharm 2017;74:1336–52.
24. Day SR, Smith D, Harris K, et al. An infectious diseases physician-led antimicrobial stewardship program at a small community hospital associated with improved susceptibility patterns and cost-savings after the first year. Open Forum Infect Dis 2015;2:ofv064.
25. Waters CD. Pharmacist-driven antimicrobial stewardship program in an institution without infectious diseases physician support. Am J Health Syst Pharm 2015;72: 466–8.
26. Pasquale TR, Trienski TL, Olexia DE, et al. Impact of an antimicrobial stewardship program on patients with acute bacterial skin and skin structure infections. Am J Health Syst Pharm 2014;71:1136–9.
27. DiDiodato G, McAthur L. Transition from a dedicated to a non-dedicated, ward-based pharmacist antimicrobial stewardship programme model in a non-academic hospital and its impact on length of stay of patients admitted with pneumonia: a prospective observational study. BMJ Open Qual 2017;6.
28. Leung V, Gill S, Sauve J, et al. Growing a "positive culture" of antimicrobial stewardship in a community hospital. Can J Hosp Pharm 2011;64:314–20.
29. Bartlett JM, Siola PL. Implementation and first-year results of an antimicrobial stewardship program at a community hospital. Am J Health Syst Pharm 2014; 71:943–9.
30. Libertin CR, Watson SH, Tillett WL, et al. Dramatic effects of a new antimicrobial stewardship program in a rural community hospital. Am J Infect Control 2017;45: 979–82.
31. Storey DF, Pate PG, Nguyen AT, et al. Implementation of an antimicrobial stewardship program on the medical-surgical service of a 100-bed community hospital. Antimicrob Resist Infect Control 2012;1:32.
32. Yam P, Fales D, Jemison J, et al. Implementation of an antimicrobial stewardship program in a rural hospital. Am J Health Syst Pharm 2012;69:1142–8.
33. Michaels K, Mahdavi M, Krug A, et al. Implementation of an antimicrobial stewardship program in a community hospital: results of a three-year analysis. Hosp Pharm 2012;47:608–16.
34. Veillette JJ, Vento T, Gelman S, et al. Implementation of a centralized telehealth-based antimicrobial stewardship program (ASP) for 16 small community hospitals (SCHs). Open Forum Infect Dis 2017;4:S278–9.

35. Krey SC, Waise J, Skrupky LP. Confronting the challenge of beta-lactam allergies: a quasi-experimental study assessing impact of pharmacy-led interventions. J Pharm Pract 2017. https://doi.org/10.1177/0897190017743154. 897190017743154.

36. Schabas A, Fisman DN, Schabas R. Control of *Clostridium difficile*-associated diarrhea by antibiotic stewardship in a small community hospital. Can J Infect Dis Med Microbiol 2012;23:82–3.

37. Vettese N, Hendershot J, Irvine M, et al. Outcomes associated with a thrice-weekly antimicrobial stewardship programme in a 253-bed community hospital. J Clin Pharm Ther 2013;38:401–4.

38. Pulcini C, Morel CM, Tacconelli E, et al. Human resources estimates and funding for antibiotic stewardship teams are urgently needed. Clin Microbiol Infect 2017; 23:785–7.

39. Srinivasan A. Engaging hospitalists in antimicrobial stewardship: the CDC perspective. J Hosp Med 2011;6(Suppl 1):S31–3.

40. Mack MR, Rohde JM, Jacobsen D, et al. Engaging hospitalists in antimicrobial stewardship: lessons from a multihospital collaborative. J Hosp Med 2016;11: 576–80.

41. Arora S, Geppert CM, Kalishman S, et al. Academic health center management of chronic diseases through knowledge networks: project ECHO. Acad Med 2007;82:154–60.

42. Davis S, Newcomer D, Bhayani N. Development and evolution of a 24-hour pharmacist-coordinated antimicrobial stewardship service in a community hospital. Hosp Pharm 2014;49:685–8.

43. Pammett RT, Ridgewell A. Development of an antimicrobial stewardship program in a rural and remote health authority. Can J Hosp Pharm 2016;69:333–4.

44. Wald H, Hulett T, Kneper B, et al. Colorado's statewide antimicrobial stewardship (AMS) collaborative final results: facilitating syndrome-specific interventions for skin and soft tissue infection (SSTI) and urinary tract infection (UTI). IDWeek 20172017. October 7, 2017.

45. Laible BR, Nazir J, Assimacopoulos AP, et al. Implementation of a pharmacist-led antimicrobial management team in a community teaching hospital: use of pharmacy residents and pharmacy students in a prospective audit and feedback approach. J Pharm Pract 2010;23:531–5.

46. Lee TC, Frenette C, Jayaraman D, et al. Antibiotic self-stewardship: trainee-led structured antibiotic time-outs to improve antimicrobial use. Ann Intern Med 2014;161:S53–8.

47. Garcell HG, Arias AV, Sandoval CP, et al. Impact of a focused antimicrobial stewardship program in adherence to antibiotic prophylaxis and antimicrobial consumption in appendectomies. J Infect Public Health 2017;10:415–20.

48. Pogue JM, Potoski BA, Postelnick M, et al. Bringing the "power" to Cerner's PowerChart for antimicrobial stewardship. Clin Infect Dis 2014;59:416–24.

49. Calloway S, Akilo HA, Bierman K. Impact of a clinical decision support system on pharmacy clinical interventions, documentation efforts, and costs. Hosp Pharm 2013;48:744–52.

50. Huber SR, Fullas F, Nelson KR, et al. retrospective evaluation of pharmacist interventions on use of antimicrobials using a clinical surveillance software in a small community hospital. Pharmacy (Basel) 2016;4.

51. LaRocco A Jr. Concurrent antibiotic review programs–a role for infectious diseases specialists at small community hospitals. Clin Infect Dis 2003;37:742–3.

52. Ohl CA, Dodds Ashley ES. Antimicrobial stewardship programs in community hospitals: the evidence base and case studies. Clin Infect Dis 2011;53(Suppl 1):S23–8 [quiz S9–30].

53. Perozziello A, Routelous C, Charani E, et al. The experiences and perspectives of implementing antimicrobial stewardship in five French hospitals: a qualitative study. Int J Antimicrob Agents 2018. https://doi.org/10.1016/j.ijantimicag.2018. 01.002.

54. Powell N, Franklin BD, Jacklin A, et al. Omitted doses as an unintended consequence of a hospital restricted antibacterial system: a retrospective observational study. J Antimicrob Chemother 2015;70:3379–83.

55. Lambl BB, Kaufman N, Kurowski J, et al. Does electronic stewardship work? J Am Med Inform Assoc 2017;24:981–5.

56. Stenehjem E, Hersh AL, Buckel WR, et al. Stewardship in community hospitals—optimizing outcomes and resources (SCORE): a cluster-randomized controlled trial investigating the impact of antibiotic stewardship in 15 small, community hospitals. Open Forum Infect Dis 2016;3:1696.

57. Moehring RW, Anderson DJ, Cochran RL, et al. Expert consensus on metrics to assess the impact of patient-level antimicrobial stewardship interventions in acute-care settings. Clin Infect Dis 2017;64:377–83.

58. Morris AM. Antimicrobial stewardship programs: appropriate measures and metrics to study their impact. Curr Treat Options Infect Dis 2014;6:101–12.

59. Akpan MR, Ahmad R, Shebl NA, et al. A review of quality measures for assessing the impact of antimicrobial stewardship programs in hospitals. Antibiotics (Basel) 2016;5. https://doi.org/10.3390/antibiotics5010005.

60. Dik JW, Hendrix R, Poelman R, et al. Measuring the impact of antimicrobial stewardship programs. Expert Rev Anti Infect Ther 2016;14:569–75.

61. Fridkin SK, Srinivasan A. Implementing a strategy for monitoring inpatient antimicrobial use among hospitals in the United States. Clin Infect Dis 2014;58:401–6.

62. Antibiotic prescribing and use in hospitals and long-term care: implementation resources. 2018. Available at: https://www.cdc.gov/antibiotic-use/healthcare/implementation.html. Accessed February 1, 2018.

63. Dimple P, Conan M. How to make antimicrobial stewardship work: practical considerations for hospitals of all sizes. Hosp Pharm 2010;45:10–21.

64. Box MJ, Sullivan EL, Ortwine KN, et al. Outcomes of rapid identification for gram-positive bacteremia in combination with antibiotic stewardship at a community-based hospital system. Pharmacotherapy 2015;35:269–76.

65. Trautner BW, Prasad P, Grigoryan L, et al. Protocol to disseminate a hospital-site controlled intervention using audit and feedback to implement guidelines concerning inappropriate treatment of asymptomatic bacteriuria. Implement Sci 2018;13:16.

66. Defining rural population. 2017. Available at: https://www.hrsa.gov/rural-health/about-us/definition/index.html. Accessed February 1, 2018.

67. Stenehjem E, Hyun DY, Septimus E, et al. Antibiotic stewardship in small hospitals: barriers and potential solutions. Clin Infect Dis 2017;65:691–6.

Role of the Pharmacist in Antimicrobial Stewardship

Diane M. Parente, PharmD[a],*, Jacob Morton, PharmD, MBA, BCPS[b]

KEYWORDS

- Pharmacist • Pharmacy • Antimicrobial stewardship
- Prospective audit with intervention and feedback • Outpatient • Long-term care
- Hospital

KEY POINTS

- Improving patient outcomes and minimizing consequences of antibiotic use should be the primary goal of antimicrobial stewardship.
- Pharmacists are core members of the antimicrobial stewardship team and assist in appropriate antimicrobial utilization, including but not limited to, prospective audit with intervention and feedback, education, development and tracking of metrics, rapid diagnostic testing, and the establishment of policies and protocols related to antimicrobials and infectious diseases.
- As part of prospective audit with intervention and feedback, pharmacists should look for patients who may benefit from infectious disease consultation, which has been shown to reduce mortality in a wide variety of infectious diseases.
- The role of a pharmacist has expanded and is vital in achieving the goals of antimicrobial stewardship programs throughout the continuum of care, including inpatient, outpatient, and long-term care sectors.
- Pharmacists are well positioned to serve as champions for ensuring regulatory requirements are met for antimicrobial stewardship, given the frequent multidisciplinary collaboration required on a daily basis.

INTRODUCTION

Stewardship, as a general concept, is defined as the "careful and responsible management of something entrusted to one's care."[1] When applied to antimicrobials, which include antibiotics, antivirals, and antifungals, health care professionals are tasked with using these agents responsibly and finding the balance between optimal effectiveness and development of resistance and toxicity. Along with infectious

Disclosure Statement: The authors have nothing to disclose.
[a] Infectious Diseases and Antimicrobial Stewardship, Department of Pharmacy, The Miriam Hospital, 164 Summit Avenue, Providence, RI 02906, USA; [b] Infectious Diseases, Department of Pharmacy, Saint Vincent Hospital, 123 Summer Street, Worcester, MA 01608, USA
* Corresponding author.
E-mail address: dgomes5@lifespan.org

diseases (ID) physicians, pharmacists are core members of the antimicrobial steward-ship (AMS) team and are champions for appropriate antimicrobial use.[2] Antimicrobial stewardship strategies used by pharmacists vary according to available resources and level of care, but may include antibiotic intravenous to oral conversions, prospective audit with intervention and feedback, pharmacokinetic and pharmacodynamic dose optimization, implementation of rapid diagnostic testing, and antibiotic preauthorization.[2] Additionally, pharmacists are the ideal health care professionals to develop protocols and procedures designed to improve antimicrobial use, given their frequent multidisciplinary interactions and committee involvement. Pharmacists also serve in a wide variety of settings, including the inpatient, ambulatory, and long-term care settings. As antimicrobials are prescribed in all of these settings, pharmacists have the opportunity to optimize these regimens as the medication expert on the patient care team. This article discusses in detail the role of the pharmacist as the medication expert in AMS activities in the inpatient and long-term care settings with a focus on clinical interventions and meeting regulatory standards for AMS.

ACCOMPLISHING ANTIMICROBIAL STEWARDSHIP ENDPOINTS

The overarching endpoints of AMS may be divided into primary and secondary goals. Optimization of patient outcomes, preventing antimicrobial resistance, and minimizing adverse events from antimicrobials may be considered primary goals of stewardship as they are directed toward the improvement of the patient and society. Focusing solely on costs may lead to use of suboptimal or more toxic antimicrobials that may increase length of hospitalization and the risk of adverse events and decrease resolution of infection. Pharmacists may accomplish both primary and secondary outcomes by reviewing antimicrobial regimens on a regular basis.[2] Four primary areas of focus during the review include the diagnosis, drug, dose, and duration. Through optimized antimicrobial regimens, shorter durations, and avoidance of antimicrobials when they are not needed, patient outcomes may be improved and cost savings may be achieved.[2]

PROSPECTIVE AUDIT WITH INTERVENTION AND FEEDBACK

The Infectious Diseases Society of America, Society for Healthcare Epidemiology of America, and the Centers for Disease Control and Prevention (CDC) have identified prospective audit with intervention and feedback (PAIF) as a core strategy of AMS programs (ASPs).[2] The goal of PAIF is aimed at improving antibiotic use while minimizing unintended consequences (eg, adverse effects, bacterial resistance, *Clostridium difficile* infection) in real time. This core strategy involves a review of patients on antimicrobial therapy to assess for appropriateness with regard to indication, drug selection, dose, route, and duration. Signs and symptoms of infection should be consistent with the indicated diagnosis. The antimicrobial selected should target the most likely bacteria, fungi, or viruses implicated in the diagnosis, and also should be dosed according to pharmacokinetic and pharmacodynamics parameters. Last, review of duration is essential, as many infections may be treated with shorter durations based on multiple studies that have identified no difference in patient outcomes when compared with longer courses of treatment.[3]

Once the patient has been thoroughly assessed, suggested changes to antimicrobial regimens and feedback are then relayed to the treating provider via a notification placed in the patient's medical record or direct verbal communication. Audits with intervention and feedback are typically completed by a clinical pharmacist, preferably with formal ID or AMS training. Although the structure of PAIF can vary depending on the health care setting and available resources, the most common approaches are 1-step and 2-step methods.[4] With a 1-step approach, a trained pharmacist audits patients on antimicrobial therapy and provides feedback to providers without the assistance of an ID physician. However, an ID physician may be available to the pharmacist to discuss more complex cases on an as-needed basis. A 2-step method consists of the pharmacist completing the audit and then presenting cases with possible interventions to the ID physician for approval before making a recommendation to the treating provider.

There are a variety of strategies pharmacists use to identify patients to prospectively audit. Patient selection for PAIF can be targeted to specific infections such as respiratory tract infections or urinary tract infections, patient location (medical or intensive care unit) where antimicrobial use may be particularly high, specific antibiotics identified via consumption data (eg, restricted, broad-spectrum, high-use, costly, or potentially toxic antibiotics), or by culture results. Interventions made by pharmacists may include antimicrobial de-escalation or broadening of antimicrobial spectrum, discontinuation, drug, dose, or duration optimization, intravenous to oral conversion, ID consultation, therapeutic drug monitoring including ordering of pertinent laboratory tests, identification of drug-drug interactions, and unnecessary duplicate antimicrobial coverage.

An advantage of PAIF is that providers can preserve their prescribing autonomy, as the acceptance of recommendations is voluntary.[2] The feedback mechanism also allows pharmacists to educate providers at the time the intervention is made. Through PAIF, pharmacists are also able to provide individualized therapy to meet patient needs and may conduct PAIF at various points through the course of a patient's antimicrobial therapy. However, PAIF can be labor-intensive for pharmacists in terms of time for review, communication of recommendations, and documentation of interventions. This may be particularly challenging in large health care settings with a high volume of patients for audit, limited time dedicated to PAIF due to a pharmacist's competing priorities, or limited pharmacist personnel to conduct and track PAIF. Pharmacists play a major role in PAIF from performing PAIF, to documenting interventions, and analyzing data to identify targets to maximize interventions that positively impact patient outcomes and improve antibiotic use.

Another major benefit of PAIF is the opportunity for pharmacists to identify patients who may benefit from an ID consultation. ID consultation is associated with decreased mortality and hospital readmission and is beneficial in patients with bacterial, fungal, and viral infections.[5–7] In patients with multiple comorbidities, those at risk for multidrug-resistant organisms, or those with complex infectious processes, the expertise provided by an ID physician assists with developing a comprehensive patient history, diagnostic considerations, and treatment strategies. Pharmacists, as part of PAIF, are able to identify these challenging patients and recommend ID involvement. A recent study of hospitalized Veterans Affairs patients demonstrated that the implementation of an ASP that used PAIF was associated with an increase in ID consultation as well as an increase in ID consultation within 48 hours of hospital admission.[8]

TRANSITIONS OF CARE WITH ANTIMICROBIALS

AMS efforts have primarily focused on improving antimicrobial use during a patient's hospitalization; however, patients often complete most of their antimicrobial course following discharge.[9–12] Although inpatient ASPs have shown to be successful, approximately two-thirds of oral antimicrobials prescribed to patients on hospital discharge were inappropriate, according to data from 2 single-center retrospective studies.[13,14] Antimicrobials prescribed at discharge were considered inappropriate based on indication, duration, spectrum, dose, and frequency.

A recent single-center, quasi-experimental, retrospective cohort study examined the impact of an institutional guidance for oral step-down antimicrobial selection and duration with a pharmacist audit of discharge prescriptions with real-time recommendations to providers.[14] The intervention resulted in a significant reduction in antimicrobial prescriptions with broad gram-negative coverage (51% to 40%), specifically with fluoroquinolones (38% to 25%). Although the total duration of therapy was not significantly lower, the duration of prescribed antimicrobials at discharge was. There was a 14% increase in overall appropriateness of antimicrobials and a significant improvement in antimicrobial selection (72% to 90%). The greatest impact of these interventions was observed in a subgroup of 289 cases of community-acquired pneumonia, urinary tract infection, and skin infections. These findings, along with those from another retrospective study, highlight these 3 infections as targets for high-yield interventions.[13] The study also examined the impact of the pharmacist's audit and feedback on discharge prescriptions. Of the 918 patients prescribed antimicrobials at discharge, 363 (40%) of the cases were reviewed by a pharmacist. As part of the PAIF, the pharmacist contacted the provider in 27% of reviewed cases and recommended to modify therapy in 86% with a 67% acceptance rate. The most common interventions made by the pharmacist were to optimize antibiotic selection, dose, and/or reduce treatment duration. In terms of patient outcomes, there were no significant differences between the preintervention and postintervention groups in incidence of treatment failure (15% vs 15%) or readmission for the same infection (8% vs 8%). Although not statistically significant, there was a lower incidence of C difficile infection (2% vs 0%) and adverse effects (7% vs 3%).

The presence of an AMS pharmacist at the transition from inpatient to outpatient care may be essential to limiting overall inappropriate antimicrobial use while curbing unintended consequences to patients. Interventions at transitions of care should focus on reducing inappropriate antimicrobial prescriptions without an acceptable indication, and those with inappropriate duration or antibiotic spectrum of activity.

LONG-TERM CARE AND OUTPATIENT SETTINGS

The inappropriate use of antimicrobials is not unique to the hospital setting. According to the CDC, up to 70% of nursing home residents receive 1 or more antibiotic courses annually.[15] Unfortunately, up to 75% of antimicrobials prescribed in long-term care settings are either incorrect or unnecessary.[16] In addition, antimicrobial utilization in the outpatient setting has shown to contribute to patient adverse events, antimicrobial resistance, health care expenditures, morbidity, and mortality.[17–20] Of most concern, antimicrobials prescribed in the outpatient setting continue to be for conditions that typically do not merit antimicrobial therapy.[21] The 2014 White House Administration issued an Executive Order to Combat Antibiotic-Resistant Bacteria, which calls for implementation of ASPs across the continuum of care, including long-term care facilities and outpatient office-based settings.[22]

Currently, limited published evidence exists for determining AMS strategies that yield impactful and sustainable interventions in the outpatient and long-term care settings. The factors that drive antibiotic misuse or overprescribing in outpatient and long-term care settings are multifactorial, and intervening in these areas is complex. Unlike the hospital setting, implementation of AMS strategies can pose a challenge as the provider, pharmacist, and patients are not always present in the same location.

However, the role of pharmacists in AMS is not limited to the inpatient sector and their skillset is valuable in achieving the goals of outpatient and long-term care ASPs.

Pharmacists have developed a presence in physician-based offices and long-term care facilities to provide medication management services. Such pharmacists have the ability to undertake the role of ASP champions if given additional AMS training. Several infectious disease pharmacy organizations offer training programs in ASP including the Society of Infectious Diseases Pharmacists and Making a Difference in Infectious Diseases. In office-based and long-term care sectors, pharmacists can assist with education on appropriate antimicrobial prescribing and resistance. Pharmacist-delivered education can be used in a variety of ways, including multidisciplinary collaboration with the formulation of local guidelines, participation in academic detailing, continuing education programs to providers and nurses, and patient education. Pharmacists can also assist in reporting of antimicrobial prescribing rates to target high-yield interventions. In addition, pharmacists with AMS training are able to conduct antimicrobial regimen reviews to make interventions on discontinuation, duration, de-escalation, and dose or frequency optimization. Further, in outpatient office-based settings, pharmacists can assist prescribers on antimicrobial need and selection. Another opportunity to optimize AMS is with point-of-care (POC) testing for IDs in community pharmacies and ambulatory settings, including office-based practices. The use of POC testing would assist in the decision to use or select an appropriate antimicrobial. Several studies have shown the benefits of using POC testing for influenza and group A streptococcal pharyngitis in both community pharmacies and ambulatory settings with no negative outcomes noted.[23,24]

Although the CDC has released Core Elements of Outpatient Antibiotic Stewardship to guide those expanding AMS practices to the outpatient realm, the literature available is still limited on identifying the most impactful practices to implement. Pharmacists have roles in several outpatient settings, including long-term care, physician offices, and community pharmacy. However, more data are needed to delineate their role and the resources needed to overcome the present barriers.

CONCORDANCE WITH REGULATORY REQUIREMENTS

Although AMS has long been recommended as best practice, attempts to standardize this best practice have been lacking until recently.[2] The Centers for Medicare and Medicaid Services proposed a rule in 2016 requiring AMS in hospital settings as a condition of participation, and was further expanded to include nursing facilities in 2017.[25,26] Beginning January 1, 2017, The Joint Commission also mandated AMS in all acute care hospitals, critical access hospitals, and nursing facilities.[27] Currently there are 7 Elements of Performance (EPs) for hospitals and 8 EPs for nursing homes. These include leadership support for stewardship, education of hospital or facility staff and practitioners regarding AMS and resistance, establishment of a multidisciplinary team that ideally includes a physician and pharmacist trained in ID, incorporation of all CDC Core Elements of Antimicrobial Stewardship into the stewardship program, development of organization-specific protocols and policies to guide appropriate antibiotic use, tracking and reporting data related to AMS efforts, and development of action plans to improve antimicrobial use in response to areas of opportunity identified through stewardship.[27] In addition, nursing facilities must also provide education to residents and their families regarding AMS and antibiotic resistance.[28]

As previously mentioned, pharmacists are identified as key members of the AMS team.[2,27] The Society for Infectious Disease Pharmacists notes that every pharmacist plays a role in AMS, even if the pharmacist is not formally trained in ID.[29] This may involve utilization of hospital protocols and procedures to initiate switching patients from intravenous to oral antibiotics to facilitate hospital discharge, de-escalating antibiotics, or other institution-specific protocols to guide antibiotic use. Furthermore, the American Society for Health System Pharmacists provides specific guidance on the responsibilities of pharmacists in AMS. As part of this guidance, pharmacists are called to be leaders within the health system by encouraging interdisciplinary collaboration, participating in the institution's pharmacy and therapeutics committee, using clinical decision-support software as part of patient care activities and data collection, and providing education to all health care professionals, patients, and family members.[30] Because pharmacists' responsibilities are so heavily dependent on interdisciplinary collaboration and incorporating all areas of patient care into their daily activities, pharmacists are well positioned to ensure that all EPs for AMS are met for accreditation purposes.

SUMMARY

Pharmacists play a vital role in the establishment and implementation of ASPs across inpatient and outpatient settings. Through regular review of antibiotic regimens as part of PAIF, pharmacists have the opportunity to optimize antimicrobial selection, dose, and duration. Furthermore, pharmacists have the necessary skills to track and report AMS metrics, in addition to ensuring all regulatory requirements are met for accreditation and reimbursement purposes. As antibiotic resistance continues to be a challenge in effectively managing patients with IDs, pharmacists will be key members of the team responsible for preserving our limited antimicrobial armamentarium.

REFERENCES

1. Stewardship. Merriam-Webster. Available at: https://www.merriam-webster.com/dictionary/stewardship. Accessed April 21, 2018.
2. Barlam TF, Cosgrove SE, Abbo LM, et al. Implementing an antibiotic stewardship program: guidelines by the Infectious Diseases Society of America and the Society for Healthcare Epidemiology of America. Clin Infect Dis 2016;62(10):e51–77.
3. Spellberg B. The new antibiotic mantra-"shorter is better". JAMA Intern Med 2016; 176(9):1254–5.
4. Chung GW, Wu JE, Yeo CL, et al. Antimicrobial stewardship: a review of prospective audit and feedback systems and an objective evaluation of outcomes. Virulence 2013;4(2):151–7.
5. Hamandi B, Husain S, Humar A, et al. Impact of infectious disease consultation on the clinical and economic outcomes of solid organ transplant recipients admitted for infectious complications. Clin Infect Dis 2014;59(8):1074–82.
6. Spec A, Olsen MA, Raval K, et al. Impact of infectious diseases consultation on mortality of cryptococcal infection in patients without HIV. Clin Infect Dis 2017; 64(5):558–64.
7. Burnham JP, Olsen MA, Stwalley D, et al. Infectious diseases consultation reduces 30-day and 1-year all-cause mortality for multidrug-resistant organism infections. Open Forum Infect Dis 2018;5(3):ofy026.
8. Morrill HJ, Gaitanis MM, LaPlante KL. Antimicrobial stewardship program prompts increased and earlier infectious diseases consultation. Antimicrob Resist Infect Control 2014;3:12.
9. Avdic E, Cushinotto LA, Hughes AH, et al. Impact of an antimicrobial stewardship intervention on shortening the duration of therapy for community-acquired pneumonia. Clin Infect Dis 2012;54(11):1581–7.

10. Jenkins TC, Knepper BC, Sabel AL, et al. Decreased antibiotic utilization after implementation of a guideline for inpatient cellulitis and cutaneous abscess. Arch Intern Med 2011;171(12):1072–9.

11. Jenkins TC, Stella SA, Cervantes L, et al. Targets for antibiotic and healthcare resource stewardship in inpatient community-acquired pneumonia: a comparison of management practices with national guideline recommendations. Infection 2013;41(1):135–44.

12. Yogo N, Haas MK, Knepper BC, et al. Antibiotic prescribing at the transition from hospitalization to discharge: a target for antibiotic stewardship. Infect Control Hosp Epidemiol 2015;36(4):474–8.

13. Scarpato SJ, Timko DR, Cluzet VC, et al. An evaluation of antibiotic prescribing practices upon hospital discharge. Infect Control Hosp Epidemiol 2017;38(3): 353–5.

14. Yogo N, Shihadeh K, Young H, et al. Intervention to reduce broad-spectrum antibiotics and treatment durations prescribed at the time of hospital discharge: a novel stewardship approach. Infect Control Hosp Epidemiol 2017;38(5):534–41.

15. Lim CJ, Kong DC, Stuart RL. Reducing inappropriate antibiotic prescribing in the residential care setting: current perspectives. Clin Interv Aging 2014;9:165–77.

16. Nicolle LE, Bentley DW, Garibaldi R, et al. Antimicrobial use in long-term-care facilities. SHEA long-term-care committee. Infect Control Hosp Epidemiol 2000; 21(8):537–45.

17. Bourgeois FT, Mandl KD, Valim C, et al. Pediatric adverse drug events in the outpatient setting: an 11-year national analysis. Pediatrics 2009;124(4):e744–50.

18. Owens RC Jr, Donskey CJ, Gaynes RP, et al. Antimicrobial-associated risk factors for *Clostridium difficile* infection. Clin Infect Dis 2008;46(Suppl 1):S19–31.

19. Shehab N, Patel PR, Srinivasan A, et al. Emergency department visits for antibiotic-associated adverse events. Clin Infect Dis 2008;47(6):735–43.

20. Centers for Disease Control and Prevention. Antibiotic resistance threats in the United States, 2013. Available at: https://www.cdc.gov/drugresistance/pdf/ar-threats-2013-508.pdf. Accessed April 18, 2018.

21. Shapiro DJ, Hicks LA, Pavia AT, et al. Antibiotic prescribing for adults in ambulatory care in the USA, 2007-09. J Antimicrob Chemother 2014;69(1):234–40.

22. Combating antibiotic resistant bacteria in September 2014. Executive Order 13676, 79 CFR 56931, 2014. Available at: https://obamawhitehouse.archives. gov/the-press-office/2014/09/18/executive-order-combating-antibiotic-resistant-bacteria. Accessed June 1, 2018.

23. Klepser DG, Klepser ME, Dering-Anderson AM, et al. Community pharmacist-physician collaborative streptococcal pharyngitis management program. J Am Pharm Assoc (2003) 2016;56(3):323–9.e1.

24. Thornley T, Marshall G, Howard P, et al. A feasibility service evaluation of screening and treatment of group A streptococcal pharyngitis in community pharmacies. J Antimicrob Chemother 2016;71(11):3293–9.

25. Centers for Medicare and Medicaid Services. CMS issues proposed rule that prohibits discrimination, reduces hospital-acquired conditions, and promotes antibiotic stewardship in hospitals. Available at: https://www.cms.gov/Newsroom/MediaReleaseDatabase/Fact-sheets/2016-Fact-sheets-items/2016-06-13.html. Accessed April 21, 2018.

26. Centers for Medicare and Medicaid Services. Final rule to reform the requirements for long-term care facilities. Available at: https://www.cms.gov/Outreach-and-Education/Outreach/NPC/Downloads/2016-10-27-LTC-Presentation.pdf. Accessed April 21, 2018.

27. The Joint Commission. The Joint Commission E-dition. Accreditation Requirements: Medication Management. Available at: https://e-dition.jcrinc.com/MainContent. aspx. Accessed April 21, 2018.
28. The Joint Commission. Accreditation and Certification. EP deletion: MM.09.01.01, EP 3 going away. Available at: https://www.jointcommission.org/issues/article. aspx?Article=YorQ4E0NZh1SOmOxW2H%2FtFFcVyCrphOFlmQsZM%2BlvPc% 3D. Accessed April 21, 2018.
29. Heil EL, Kuti JL, Bearden DT, et al. The essential role of pharmacists in antimicrobial stewardship. Infect Control Hosp Epidemiol 2016;37(7):753–4.
30. ASHP statement on the pharmacist's role in antimicrobial stewardship and infection prevention and control. Am J Health Syst Pharm 2010;67(7):575–7.

The Pharmacoeconomic Aspects of Antibiotic Stewardship Programs

Cheston B. Cunha, MD

KEYWORDS

- Antimicrobial stewardship • Pharmacoeconomics • Oral antibiotic therapy • Cost

KEY POINTS

- Antibiotic stewardship programs offer significant cost saving to institutions and will ultimately pay for themselves.
- Interventions with the highest cost-saving focus on intravenous to oral and oral-only therapy.
- Certain therapies that may seem less costly at first look may hold hidden costs (both direct and indirect) that actually make them less desirable options.

INTRODUCTION

The objective of antimicrobial stewardship programs (ASPs) is to promote optimal use of antimicrobial therapy. Optimal antibiotic use is based on several factors that vary in importance depending on the patient and hospital area.[1–3] The traditional basis of selection takes into account the following:

1. Antibiotic spectrum (appropriate for the usual pathogens that are site-dependent)
2. Tissue penetration (drug must reach site of infection in therapeutic concentrations)
3. Resistance potential (use in an individual case may be effective, but depending on the antibiotic, may also induce resistance)
4. Good safety profile (few infrequent serious side effects)
5. Should be relatively cost-effective (vs alternatives)

PHARMACOECOMONIC PERSPECTIVE

Pharmacoeconomics of antimicrobial therapy must take into account the above-mentioned factors, and appropriately, cost is usually not the most important factor in antibiotic selection. The least expensive drug is usually accompanied by

Antibiotic Stewardship Program, Division of Infectious Disease, Rhode Island Hospital, 593 Eddy Street, Physicians Office Building, Suite #328, Providence, RI 02903, USA
E-mail address: ccunha@Lifespan.org

Med Clin N Am 102 (2018) 937–946
https://doi.org/10.1016/j.mcna.2018.05.010
0025-7125/18/© 2018 Elsevier Inc. All rights reserved.
medical.theclinics.com

other concerns, such as high resistance potential, poor side effect profile, pharmacokinetic (PK) properties that limit penetration into target tissue (site of infection), and/or suboptimal activity against the presumed/known pathogen. It is false economy to preferentially select the least expensive antibiotics solely because of its cost.[2–4] It is false economy and not good for ASPs, if the inexpensive antibiotic selected fails or causes resistance problems (in other patients/hospitals). Therapeutic failure, in the end, requires retreatment with a more costly, but effective antibiotic.[2,5]

ANTIBIOTIC PHARMACOKINETIC COST DETERMINANTS

Antibiotic costs depend on several cost determining factors, which when combined are the basis of antibiotic cost to the hospital/patient. The first cost factor is acquisition cost to the hospital or patient cost from the pharmacy.[2,3] Because the main thrust of ASP is in hospital, this article primarily focuses on inpatient aspects; added to the cost of the antibiotic is the cost to the hospital of administering the drug intravenously (IV). Obviously, with oral (PO) there is only acquisition cost and no cost for IV administration.[2,6] The average wholesale price is used for comparative purposes but varies considerably (volume discounts) among hospitals, buying groups, and consortia.

Generally, acceptance of administering an IV dose of antibiotic is $10/dose. This cost includes pharmacy costs of storage, labeling/dispensing, and IV administration (diluent, syringes/bags) and IV team or nursing time to administer the IV formulation (**Box 1**).

Obviously, the cost of daily administration may exceed, in cases of inexpensive antibiotics, the acquisition cost of the antibiotic, eg, IV ampicillin q4h costs $60/day to administer which is in excess (and must be added to) the acquisition cost of the drug. Therefore, the actual cost to the hospital of an antibiotic with a short half-life (t ½) may be more expensive when added administrative costs are factored in.[7,8]

OTHER ANTIBIOTIC COST DETERMINANTS

As mentioned earlier, an antibiotic with suboptimal activity or spectrum and suboptimal PK characteristics that prevent penetration at the infection site frequently fail and require retreatment cost multiplier.[3,5,7] There is also a hidden cost of inducing resistance. Treating multidrug-resistant organisms (MDROs) usually requires expensive antibiotics. It is difficult to assess this factor in ASP programs but is a daily problem in the inpatient and outpatient settings. Every effort should be made to use "low resistance potential" antibiotics; only those with a "high resistance potential" should be used to minimize the emergence of resistance among Gram-negative bacilli (GNB).

The acquisition cost plus the IV administration cost may be modest but often results in the more expensive and clinically difficult problem of trending MDR GNB infection[4,9–11] (see **Box 1**).

Other indirect cost factors include the cost of collateral damage, that is, side effects, *Clostridium difficile*, and drug-drug interactions. It is important to recognize from an ASP perspective that most antibiotics (eg, macrolide, tetracycline, aztreonam, colistin, polymyxin B, tigecycline, Q/D, nitrofurantoin, fosfomycin, and aminoglycosides) do not cause *C difficile* infection. Carbapenems and quinolones (FQ) may cause *C difficile* infection, but the antibiotics within the highest *C difficile* potential are clindamycin and the β-lactams (excluding ceftriaxone). Some

---

Box 1
Beyond antibiotic acquisition costs: the indirect costs of antibiotics

1. Cost of IV administration ($10/dose):
   a. If clinically acceptable, other things being equal, preferentially use antibiotics with *less frequent dosing intervals*;
      i. For uncomplicated streptococcal cellulitis, both cefazolin and ceftriaxone are equally effective;
   b. Acquisition drug costs aside, as cefazolin is given q8h (3 doses × $10/dose = $30/d), cefazolin *costs more to administer* than ceftriaxone given q24h (1 dose × $10/dose = $10/d).

2. Cost of obligatory other drug with "double drug" therapy:
   a. For intraabdominal infections (IAIs): metronidazole *plus another antiaerobic Gram-negative bacillus antibiotic* = the actual cost of using metronidazole for IAIs;
   b. Community-acquired pneumonia (CAP): ceftriaxone *plus azithromycin* = the actual cost of using ceftriaxone for CAP.

3. Cost of monitoring:
   a. Serial serum creatinine determinations to monitor renal dysfunction and to calculate creatinine clearances;
   b. Liver function tests to monitor hepatic drug reactions;
   c. Drug level measurements to monitor drug efficacy or toxicity.

4. Cost of antibiotic resistance from multidrug-resistant organisms (MDROs):
   a. Length of stay (LOS) up;
   b. Economic implications of suboptimal bed utilization and infection control contaminant measures;
   c. Needless treatment of bacterial colonization (vs infection), which often predisposes to MDROs;
   d. Cost of retreatment with another, usually more expensive, effective antibiotic.

5. Cost of therapeutic failure:
   a. Length of stay (LOS) up;
   b. Cost of consultants/tests to determine the cause of persistent fever on treatment;
   c. Cost of retreatment with another, usually more expensive, effective antibiotic.

6. Cost of adverse effects:
   a. Seizures;
   b. Non-*Clostridium difficile* diarrhea;
   c. *C difficile* diarrhea/colitis;
   d. Phlebitis;
   e. Drug fever;
   f. Drug rashes;
   g. Hypersensitivity reactions (anaphylaxis).

Abbreviation: IV, intravenous.

Adapted from Cunha CB. Pharmacoeconomic implications of antimicrobial adverse events. In: LaPlante KL, Cunha CB, Morrill HJ, et al, editors. Antimicrobial stewardship: principles and practice. Oxfordshire (United Kingdom): CABI Press; 2017; with permission.

---

antibiotics are actually protective against *C difficile*, for example, doxycycline and tigecycline.

It is recognized from an ASP perspective that some antibiotics are not the only drugs that may cause *C difficile* infection.[3,12,13] Frequent causes of *C difficile* infection are proton pump inhibitors (PPIs), cancer chemotherapy, and some psych medications. PPIs may cause *C difficile* infection alone or, when used with FQ or carbapenems, may distort the data suggesting a higher than actual *C difficile* incidence of FQ and carbapenems.

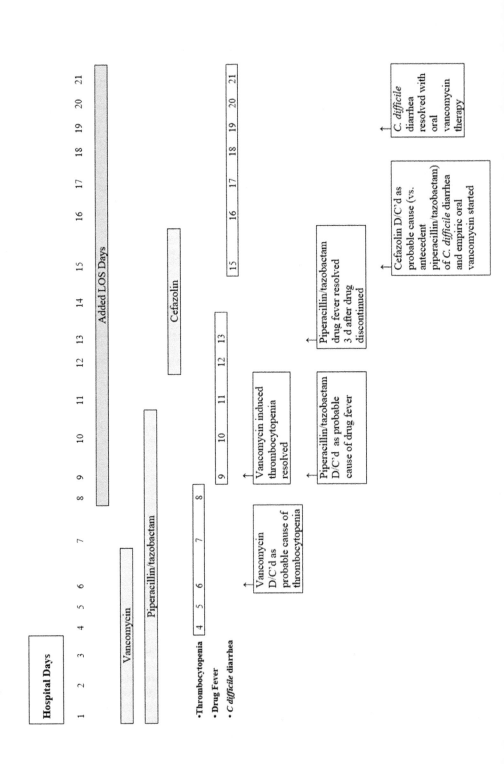

Other common cost-intensive antibiotic side effects are drug fevers and drug rashes. These diagnoses require subspecialty consultations, additional laboratory testing, and often increase in hospital length of stay (LOS)[14–19] (**Fig. 1, Table 1**).

PHARMACOECONOMIC ASP STRATEGIES

Optimal therapy begins with selecting an antibiotic with the appropriate spectrum relative to the infection site and with a high degree of activity against the usual pathogens at the infection site. Second, select an antibiotic with a "low resistance potential" and favorable side effect profile. The antibiotic should have a low *C difficile* potential. Given the general principles discussed, there are some ASP interventions that have important pharmacoeconomic implications. With IV therapy, select an antibiotic with a long t ½, which permits less frequent dosing. This reduces hospital drug administration costs.

The most important ASP intervention that also has pharmacoeconomic implication is the use of IV-to-PO switch therapy or even better PO-only therapy.[19–22] IV-to-PO therapy has been shown to be as effective as IV therapy. Switch therapy, IV to PO, has several clinical and pharmacoeconomic advantages, for example, shorter hospital LOS and earlier hospital discharges. Both of these are important for a patient, infection control, and economic perspective.[23,24] With a variety of infectious diseases, for example, CAP IV-to-PO switch therapy has been shown to be usually efficacious as IV therapy. Among ASP strategies, IV-to-PO switch programs are the "low hanging fruit" of ASP interventions with important pharmacoeconomic benefits[23–26] (**Table 2**).

If IV-to-PO switch is a useful ASP intervention then PO-only therapy is even better[6,12,27] (**Table 3**). PO-only therapy is an idea whose time has come. Now clinicians have sufficient experience and confidence with the PO portion of IV-to-PO switch therapy. The advantages of PO therapy are even greater by eliminating the IV portion of therapy.

There is a reluctance by practitioners to change habits and tend to be creatures of habit and may base their approaches on a variety of incorrect preconceptions (ie, IV therapy is more effective than PO therapy, IV therapy results in a rapid therapeutic response).

The antibiotics recommended for PO therapy are those with all the requisite properties of an IV antibiotic and in addition are well absorbed (high bioavailability >90%) so that serum/tissue concentrations are the same at any given dose. For example, with levofloxacin, moxifloxacin, doxycycline, minocycline, TMP-SMX, and linezolid, gastrointestinal (GI) absorption is greater than or equal to 90%, resulting in the same serum/tissue levels with the same IV dose as PO. GI absorption is rapid/complete such that effective serum levels are present after half an hour. In patients who are critically ill and are likely not to recover within 1 hour, the initial therapy should be IV. Even in critically ill patients who are in intensive care unit, GI antibiotic absorption is the same or enhanced when given PO (via nasogastric/percutaneous endoscopic gastrostomy tube) in shock. With shock and hypotension, there is peripheral vasoconstriction with blood preferentially shunted to vital organs (including the stomach) so that antibiotic absorption is better than without shock.

Fig. 1. Pharmacoeconomic implications of antimicrobial adverse effects on hospital costs and LOS: a schematic representation of a case of lower extremity cellulitis and potential AEs. (*Adapted from* Cunha CB. Pharmacoeconomic implications of antimicrobial adverse events. In: LaPlante KL, Cunha CB, Morrill HJ, et al, editors. Antimicrobial stewardship: principles and practice. Oxfordshire (United Kingdom): CABI Press; 2017. p. 338; with permission.)

Table 1
Pharmacoeconomic implications of antimicrobial adverse events

Antimicrobial Adverse Effects	Pharmacoeconomic Parameters		
	Economic Potential (Added Costs of Laboratory Tests, Subspecialty Consultants)	Potential for Increased LOS (Prolonged LOS with Reduced Reimbursement and Suboptimal Bed Utilization)	Medicolegal Potential (Cost of Lawsuits and Attendant Adverse Institutional Publicity and Damaged Reputation)
Drug fevers	+++	+++	−
Drug rashes	…	…	…
Maculopapular rashes	+	++	+
Stevens-Johnson syndrome	+	+++	+++
Anaphylaxis	+	−	+++
Thrombocytopenia	+	+++	++
Leukopenia	++	+	−
Anemia	+	−	+
Pancytopenia	++	+	+
Elevated transaminase	++	+	+
Interstitial nephritis	+++	++	−
Phlebitis	++	+	−
Seizures	+++	+	−
Encephalopathy	+++	++	−
Diarrhea	…	…	…
Non-*Clostridium difficile* diarrhea	+	−	−
C difficile diarrhea	++	++	+
C difficile colitis	+++	+++	+++

Abbreviations: −, little/no impact; +, minimal impact; ++, moderate impact; +++, high impact.

Table 2
Clinical and pharmacoeconomic advantages of oral antibiotic therapy

	Advantages	Comments
Oral Antibiotic therapy	Lower antibiotic acquisition cost (at same dose) No IV antibiotic administration costs ($10/dose) Rapid gastrointestinal absorption (~1 h even in critical ill patients) Eliminates phlebitis and IV line-related infections Decreases LOS Patients pleased with earlier discharge	Avoid if markedly impaired gastrointestinal absorption If therapeutic effect is needed in <1 h (patient in shock), begin therapy IV and later switch to PO to complete therapy

Table 3
Treatment cost of intravenous and oral antibiotics

IV Antibiotics	Usual Adult Dose (70 kg)	Cost per Dose	IV Admin. Cost ($10/Dose)	Drug Cost per Day	Lowest Wholesale Price per Dose (Average Wholesale Price [AWP], Where Known per Dose, as per REDBOOK 2016)
Levofloxacin	500 mg (IV) q24 h	$4.50	$10	$4.50 + $10 = $14.50	$8.45 ($24.2)
	750 mg (IV) q24 h	$7.49	$10	$7.49 + $10 = $17.49	$25.2 ($29.2)
Ciprofloxacin	400 mg (IV) q12 h	$3.44	$20	$6.88 + $20 = $26.88	$3.44 ($3.48)
Clindamycin	600 mg (IV) q8h	$5.09	$30	$15.27 + $30 = $45.27	$3.48
Linezolid	600 mg (IV) q12 h	$112.74	$20	$225.48 + $20 = $245.48	$96.00 ($599.49)
Doxycycline	100 mg (IV) q12 h	$16.80	$20	$33.60 + $20 = $53.60	$18.20
Minocycline	100 mg (IV) q12 h	$71.18	$20	$142.36 + $20 = $162.36	$65.30 ($120.89)
Metronidazole	500 mg (IV) q8h	$1.08	$30	$3.24 + $30 = $33.24	$2.34
TMP-SMX	160/800 mg (IV) q6h	$8.70	$40	$34.80 + $40 = $74.80	$5.35 ($12.73)

PO Antibiotics	Usual Adult Dose (70 kg)	Cost per Dose	IV Admin. Cost ($10/Dose)	Drug Cost per Day	AWP per Dose as per REDBOOK 2016
Levofloxacin	500 mg (PO) q24 h	$0.50	$0	$0.50	$15.60
	750 mg (PO) q24 h	$1.05	$0	$1.05	$24.60
Ciprofloxacin	500 mg (PO) q12 h	$0.11	$0	$0.22	$3.44
	750 mg (PO) q12 h	$0.35	$0	$0.70	$5.17
Clindamycin	300 mg (PO) q6h	$1.28	$0	$3.85	$1.45
Linezolid	600 mg (PO) q12 h	$111.95	$0	$223.90	$183.00
Doxycycline	100 mg (PO) q12 h	$2.37	$0	$4.74	$0.08 ($3)
Minocycline	100 mg (PO) q12 h	$0.20	$0	$0.40	$1.67
Metronidazole	500 mg (PO) q8h	$0.65	$0	$1.95	$0.69
TMP-SMX	1 DS tablet (PO) q6h	$1.15	$0	$4.60	$0.49

Costs are estimates based on average US pricing.

Adapted from Cunha CB. Pharmacoeconomic implications of antimicrobial adverse events. In: LaPlante KL, Cunha CB, Morrill HJ, et al, editors. Antimicrobial stewardship: principles and practice. Oxfordshire (United Kingdom): CABI Press; 2017; with permission.

Table 4
Antibiotic stewardship program pharmacoeconomic strategies

First Tier Strategies	Second Tier Strategies	Third Tier Strategies
• Optimize dose/dosing interval according to PK/PD principles and site of infection • If possible, select antibiotics with a low *Clostridium difficile* potential or one that is protective against *C difficile* • Avoid if possible, nonantibiotic causes of *C difficile*, for example, PPIs	• Preferentially use antibiotics with a "low resistance potential" • IV-to-PO switch program to decrease antibiotic costs and the LOS • Educate and encourage practitioners of the many clinical and pharmacoeconomic advantages of PO-only antibiotic therapy	• Use prospective adults to assess the effectiveness and cost savings of ASP interventions • Use ASP pharmacoeconomic measures to fund ASP efforts

The ASP pharmacoeconomic advantages of PO-only therapy are impressive. First, at the same dose, PO days are almost always (except linezolid) less expensive than their IV counterpart. Furthermore, there is no IV administration change with PO antibiotics. Avoiding the use of peripheral/central lines also has economic implications as it is impossible to develop phlebitis or a line infection if no line is present. Even more than with IV-to-PO switch therapy, PO-only increases patient satisfaction, decreases LOS, and permits earlier discharge to complete PO therapy at home[2,6] (**Table 4**).

SUMMARY

ASP programs are charged with optimizing antibiotic use and minimizing resistance and *C difficile*. In addition, there are important pharmacoeconomic aspects of ASP that can save hospital/health care system resources, and such savings should be used to support ASP staff and support systems.[2,28–30]

REFERENCES

1. Cunha CB. Principles of antimicrobial stewardship. In: LaPlante KL, Cunha CB, Morrill HJ, et al, editors. Antimicrobial stewardship: principles and practice. London: CABI Press; 2017. p. 1–8.
2. Cunha CB. Pharmacoeconomic implications of antimicrobial adverse events. In: LaPlante KL, Cunha CB, Morrill HJ, et al, editors. Antimicrobial stewardship: principles and practice. London: CABI Press; 2017. p. 334–41.
3. Cunha CB, Cunha BA, editors. Antibiotic essentials. 15th edition. New Delhi (India): Jay Pee Medical Publishers; 2017.
4. Cunha BA. Factors in antibiotic formulary selection: antibiotic costs. P&T 2003;28: 662–5.
5. Cunha BA, Ortega AM. Antibiotic failure. Med Clin North Am 1995;79:663–72.
6. Cunha BA. Intravenous-to-oral antibiotic switch therapy. A cost-effective approach. Postgrad Med 1997;1001:111–2.
7. Zimichman E, Henderson D, Tamir O, et al. Health care associated infections: a meta analysis of costs and financial impact of the US health care system. JAMA Intern Med 2013;173:2039–46.
8. Mertz D, Plagge H, Bassetti S, et al. How much money can be saved by applying intravenous antibiotics once instead of several times a day? Infection 2010;38: 479–82.

9. Colli A, Campodonico R, Gherli T. Early switch from vancomycin to oral linezolid for treatment of Gram positive heart valve endocarditis. Annu Thorac Surg 2007; 84:87–91.

10. Cunha BA. Effective antibiotic resistance control strategies. Lancet 2001;357: 1307–8, 358, 1101.

11. Cartaxo Salgado FX, Carneiro Goncalves J, Monteiro De Souza C, et al. Cost of antimicrobial treatment of patients infected with multidrug resistant organisms in the intensive care unit. Medicine 2011;11:531–5.

12. Bouza E. Consequences of Clostridium difficile infection: understanding the healthcare burden. Clnical Microbial Infect 2012;18:5–12.

13. McGlone SM, Bailey RR, Zimmer SM, et al. The economic burden of C. difficile. Clin Microbiol Infect 2012;18:282–9.

14. Cambell R, Dean B, Nathanson B, et al. Length of stay and hospital costs among high-risk patients with hospital origin C. difficile associateddiarrhea. J Med Econ 2013;16:440–8.

15. Roberts RR, Hota B, Ahmad I, et al. Hospital and societal costs of antimicrobial resistant infections in a Chicago teaching hospital: implications for antibiotic stewardship. Clin Infect Dis 2009;49:1175–84.

16. File TM. Duration and cessation of antimicrobial treatment. J Hosp Med 2012;7: s22–33.

17. Gray A, Dryden M, Charos A. Antibiotic management and early discharge from a hospital: an economic analysis. J Antimicrob Chemother 2012;67:2297–302.

18. Yen YH, Chen HY, Wuan Jin L, et al. Clinical and economic impact of a pharmacist managed iv to po conversion service for levofloxacin in Taiwan. Int J Clin Pharmacol Ther 2012;50:136–41.

19. Signorovitch JE, Sheng Duh M, Sengupta A, et al. Hospital visits and costs following outpatient treatment of CAP with levofloxacin or moxifloxacin. Curr Med Res Opin 2010;26:355–63.

20. Restrepo MI, Frei CR. Health economics of use of fluroquinolones to treat patients with community-acquired pneumonia. Amer J Med 2010;123(4,Suppl): S39–46.

21. Goff DA, Bauer KA, Reed EE, et al. Is the low-hanging fruit worth picking for antimicrobial stewardship programs? Clin Infect Dis 2012;55:587–92.

22. Ott SR, Hauptmeier BM, Emen C, et al. Treatment failure in pneumonia: impact of antibiotic treatment and cost analysis. Eur Respir J 2012;39:611–8.

23. Wilke MH. Multiresistant bacteria and current therapy – the economical side of the story. Eur J Med Res 2010;15:571–6.

24. Mokabberi R, Hafbaradaran A, Ravakhah K. Doxycycline vs. levofloxacin in the treatment of community acquired pneumonia. J Clin Pharm Ther 2010;35: 195–200.

25. Malani AN, Richards PG, Kapila S, et al. Clinical and economic outcomes from a community hospitals antimicrobial stewarsship program. Amer J Infect Control 2013;41:145–8.

26. Mansouri MD, Cadle RM, Agbahiwe SO, et al. Impact of an antibiotic restriction program on antibiotic utilization in the treatment of community acquired pneumonia in a Veterans Affairs Medical Center. Infection 2011;39:53–8.

27. Cunha BA. Oral antibiotic therapy of serious systemic infections. Med Clin North Am 2006;90:1197–222.

28. Cunha CB, Varghese CA, Mylonakis E. Antimicrobial stewardship programs (ASPs): the devil is in the details. Virulence 2013;4:147–9.

29. Nicolau DP. Containing costs and containing bugs: are they mutually exclusive? J Manag Care Pharm 2009;15(2 Supp):S12–7.
30. Niwa T, Shinoda Y, Suzuki A, et al. Outcome measurement of extensive implementation of antimicrobial stewardship in patients receiving intravenous antibiotics in a Japanese university hospital. Int J Clin Pract 2012;66:999–1008.

Antibiotic Stewardship Program Perspective
Oral Antibiotic Therapy for Common Infectious Diseases

Cheston B. Cunha, MD

KEYWORDS

- Antimicrobial stewardship • Antibiotics • IV-to-oral • Oral therapy
- Pharmacokinetics • Pharmacodynamics

KEY POINTS

- If chosen properly, oral therapy provides many benefits over intravenous therapy.
- Skin soft tissue infections, community-acquired pneumonia, and urinary tract infections are relatively low-hanging fruit for oral-only therapy.
- Applying pharmacokinetic and pharmacodynamic principles, oral therapy can be used to treat even severe infectious diseases.

INTRODUCTION

Traditionally, for many bacterial infectious diseases, initial antibiotic therapy was administered intravenously (IV). Over the past 3 decades, there has been increased understanding, appreciation, and application of pharmacokinetic (PK) and pharmacodynamic (PD) principles in antibiotic therapy.

The utilization of PK/PD parameters as applied to antimicrobial therapy has led to optimizing dosage regimens as well as increased awareness and experience with oral antibiotic therapy.[1,2]

The antibiotics that lend themselves to oral administration are those that are well absorbed orally such that serum/tissue levels are essentially the same IV or orally. Clearly, if an oral antibiotic, given at the same dose as its IV formulation, results in the same serum/tissue levels, why not treat with oral antibiotics whenever possible?

In recent years, there has been an evolution from predominantly IV therapy to IV-to-oral switch therapy to entirely oral therapy for noncritical inpatients as well as outpatients.[3–5]

Antibiotic Stewardship Program, Division of Infectious Disease, Rhode Island Hospital, 593 Eddy Street, Physicians Office Building, Suite #328, Providence, RI 02903, USA
E-mail address: ccunha@lifespan.org

Med Clin N Am 102 (2018) 947–954
https://doi.org/10.1016/j.mcna.2018.05.006
0025-7125/18/© 2018 Elsevier Inc. All rights reserved.

However, physicians are creatures of habit and do not readily accept change. Most doctors were trained to begin therapy via the IV route. This practice assures rapid attainment of serum/tissue levels. Certainly, in critically ill patients in danger of dying in the next half hour should receive initial antibiotic therapy IV.[3–5]

Patients are often admitted for IV antibiotic therapy, for example, osteomyelitis, as if the route of administration is of paramount importance over PK/PD considerations and resistance potential concerns.[2] Optimal therapy does not depend on the route of antibiotic administration. Even with critically ill patients in the intensive care unit, oral antibiotics administered via nasogastric tube are not only well absorbed but absorption may also be better than in noncritically ill individuals.[6–8]

Even though there is a long experience in treating some serious systemic infections exclusively with oral antibiotics, for example, plague, rocky mountain spotted fever, there persists the mistaken notion that somehow IV is more effective than oral antibiotic therapy.[9,10]

The many advantages of oral antibiotic therapy have been realized in IV-to-oral switch programs. Advantages of the oral portion of IV-to-oral switch therapy includes lower drug costs, no phlebitis, increased patient satisfaction, no peripherally inserted central catheter lines (with their associated complications of bacteremia, fungemia), earlier discharge, and decreased length of stay (LOS)[11–16] (**Table 1**).

If IV-to-oral switch is good, then entirely oral therapy is even better.[2–5] Sometimes medical practice needs prompting, and the Centers for Disease Control and Prevention's mandated antibiotic stewardship programs (ASPs) have provided the impetetus.[17–19]

Although IV-to-oral switch is a recommended part of hospital ASPs, practitioners can take ASPs to the next level by using oral antibiotic therapy whenever possible.[2,3]

There are only 2 clinical scenarios, when IV is the preferred therapy, that is, inadequate absorption, and in critically ill patients likely to die in a half hour or less.[2,5,6] Otherwise, all other patients are candidates for entirely oral antibiotic therapy. ASPs should provide practitioners with antibiotics and doses that have the relevant PK/PD properties that essentially makes oral equivalent to IV therapy (high bioavailability: 90% absorption). The equivalence of oral therapy with IV therapy is straightforward with antibiotics of the same class, that is, oral levofloxacin = IV levofloxacin (at the same dose) with the same serum/tissue levels. Using oral antibiotics with high bioavailability (>90% absorbed), oral therapy = IV therapy pharmacokineticly[1,2,20,21] (**Table 2**).

ASPs should provide guidance when no same drug oral equivalent is available, for example, ceftriaxone. The oral equivalent (same spectrum) of ceftriaxone would be levofloxacin or Trimethoprim-sulfamethoxazole (TMP-SMX).[2–4] Shortening duration

Table 1		
Clinical and pharmacoeconomic advantages of oral antibiotic therapy		
	Advantages	**Comments**
Oral antibiotic therapy	Lower *antibiotic acquisition* cost (at same dose)	Avoid if markedly impaired gastrointestinal absorption
	No *IV antibiotic administration* costs ($10/dose)	*If therapeutic effect is* needed in <1 h (patient in shock), begin therapy IV and later switch to PO to complete therapy
	Rapid gastrointestinal absorption (~1 h even in critical ill patients)	
	Eliminates phlebitis and IV line–related infections	
	Decreases LOS	
	Patients pleased with earlier discharge	

Table 2
Bioavailability of oral antimicrobials

Bioavailability	Antimicrobials		
Excellent (>90%)	Amoxicillin	TMP	Linezolid
	Cephalexin	TMP-SMX	Tedizolid
	Cefprozil	Doxycycline	Isavuconazole
	Cefadroxil	Minocycline	Voriconazole
	Clindamycin	Fluconazole	Rifampin
	Quinolones	Metronidazole	Isoniazid
	Chloramphenicol	Cycloserine	Pyrazinamide
Good (60%–90%)	Cefixime	Valacyclovir	Ethambutol
	Cefpodoxime	Famciclovir	5-Flucytosine
	Ceftibuten	Valganciclovir	Posaconazole
	Cefuroxime	Macrolides	Itraconazole (solution)
		Cefaclor	Nitazoxanide (with food)
		Nitrofurantoin	
Poor (<60%)	Vancomycin	Cefdinir	Nitazoxanide (without food)
	Acyclovir	Cefditoren	Fosfomycin

of treatment is another ASP goal for both inpatients and outpatients. Duration of course, is independent of route of administration. For years infectious disease experts in antibiotic therapy have used entirely oral therapy to treat a variety of systemic infections, for example, endocarditis[3,5] (**Table 3**). To gain physician confidence, initial efforts with entirely oral therapy should be focused to optimize results, for example, for skin soft tissue infections (SSTIs) community-acquired pneumonia (CAP), and urinary tract infections (UTIs).[12–19,22]

Table 3
Oral antibiotic therapy of selected infectious diseases

Acute Infections	Subacute/Chronic Infections
Anthrax	Q fever
Plague	Brucellosis
Tularemia	Leptospirosis
Rocky Mountain spotted fever (RMSF)	Nocardia
Typhoid fever	Actinomycosis
Legionnaire disease	Melioidosis
Diphtheria	Bartonellosis
Vibrio vulnificus	Lung abscesses[a]
Cholera	Liver abscesses[a]
Clostridium difficile	Intraabdominal abscesses[a]
Pneumocystis (jiroveci) carinii pneumonia (PCP)	Pelvis abscesses[a]
	Renal abscesses[a]
Malaria	Sinusitis
Lyme disease (neuroborreliosis, myocarditis)	Pyelonephritis
Febrile neutropenia	Prostatitis
Nosocomial pneumonia	Complicated skin/soft tissue infections (cSSTIs)
Acute bacterial endocarditis in IVDAs (MRSA)	Osteomyelitis
	Pulmonary and extrapulmonary TB

Abbreviations: IVDA, intravenous drug abusers; MRSA, methicillin-resistant *Staphylococcus aureus*; TB, tuberculosis.
[a] May also require abscess drainage.
Adapted from Cunha BA. Oral antibiotic therapy of serious systematic infections. Med Clin North Am 2006;90(6):1203; with permission.

Accordingly, in tabular form, this article focuses on cellulitis, CAP, cystitis, and skin abscesses.[2] The oral antibiotics suggested are as effective as IV equivalents, have an excellent record of efficacy, have a good side effect profile, are relatively inexpensive (compared with IV), and have a low resistance potential. It is suggested that practitioners begin or further use oral antibiotic therapy for these infections.[2,23,24] Success should encourage further use of entirely oral therapy for other clinical syndromes.

In selecting an antibiotic, several factors should be considered. Firstly, the antibiotic's spectrum should be highly active against the usual pathogens at the site of infection. For example, coverage for cellulitis should be directed against group A streptococcus (GAS)/group B streptococcus (GBS); but because cellulitis is not caused by methicillin-sensitive *Staphylococcus aureus* (MSSA)/methicillin-resistant *Staphylococcus aureus* (MRSA), coverage for these pathogens is not necessary. Similarly, in a skin abscess, MSSA or MRSA is the usual pathogen but GAS/GBS are not. Secondly, for the antibiotic to be effective, it must reach the site of infection in therapeutic concentrations. Subtherapeutic concentrations predict resistance and/or therapeutic failure; for example, antibiotic treatment of abscesses is ineffective because antibiotics cannot penetrate in sufficient concentrations to sterilize abscess contents; for this reason, abscess drainage is needed for cure. Thirdly, the antibiotic selected should have a low resistance potential to avoid inducing antibiotic resistance; for example, ampicillin is a high-resistance-potential antibiotic, whereas doxycycline is a low-resistance-potential antibiotic. Fourthly, the safety profile is important so as to avoid potential side effects; for example, *Clostridium difficile* may be more problematic than the infection being treated.

Initial-experience oral antibiotic therapy should include common clinical syndromes, that is, cellulitis/skin abscesses, CAP, and cystitis. Although many other more serious infections may be effectively treated entirely with oral antibiotics, the previously mentioned infections are a good way to begin.

Antibiotics selected for oral administration should have all the necessary properties of their IV counterparts and in addition be well absorbed (>90% bioavailability).

Because patient compliance is essential for cure, oral antibiotics should be well tolerated and have a long half-life (t ½) that determines the dosing interval. If other factors are equal, select an oral antibiotic with a long t ½ that permits once- or twice-daily dosing to enhance patient compliance.

Applying these principles to this article, that is, SSTIs, CAP, and cystitis, the antibiotics suggested are optimal choices taking into account the 4 selection factors previously mentioned. With SSTIs, the key determinant in antibiotic selection is to appreciate that cellulitis is caused by GAS/GBS but not MSSA/MRSA. For cellulitis, cephalexin is suggested. Although other longer-acting oral cephalosporins might be effective, cephalexin, given every 6 hours, has the greatest inherent activity against GAS/GBS. Abscesses, as mentioned, if well encapsulated, need incision and drainage for cure. Because MSSA and MRSA are the usual pathogens, streptococcal coverage is not required. Physicians must be careful to interpret susceptibility data correctly. Commonly, MRSA is reported susceptible to doxycycline, clindamycin, and TMP-SMX. None of these antibiotics are highly effective against MRSA, and therapeutic failure is common. For this reason, minocycline is preferred to doxycycline even though not routinely tested.[20,21,25]

There are many treatment regimens for CAP. Clinicians should be able to differentiate typical CAP for atypical CAP by the presence or absence of extrapulmonary features. With typical bacterial CAP, clinical findings are confined to the lungs, whereas with atypical CAP, there is pneumonia plus a variety of extrapulmonary findings. It is a common practice to add atypical coverage with a macrolide, for example,

Table 4
Oral antibiotic therapy of selected common clinical syndromes

Clinical Syndromes	Usual Pathogens	Nonpathogens in This Setting	Optimal Oral Therapy	Usual Dosage[a]	Usual Duration	Percent Orally Absorbed	Peak Serum Level
SSTIs							
Cellulitis	GAS GBS	MSSA MRSA	Cephalexin	1 g (PO) q8h	× 2 wk	99% (PO = IV ceftriaxone, cefazolin)	36 mcg/mL
			Levofloxacin	500 mg (PO) q24h		99% (PO = IV levofloxacin)	8 mcg/mL
			Clindamycin	300 mg (PO) q8h		90% (PO = IV clindamycin)	2.5 mcg/mL
Skin abscesses	MSSA	MRSA GAS GBS	Cephalexin	1 g (PO) q8h	2 wk	99% (PO = IV ceftriaxone, cefazolin)	36 mcg/mL
	MRSA	MSSA GAS GBS	Levofloxacin	500 mg (PO) q24h		99% (PO = IV levofloxacin)	8 mcg/mL
			Minocycline[b]	100 mg (PO) q12h	1–2 wk	95% (PO = IV minocycline)	4 mcg/mL
			Linezolid	600 mg (PO) q12h		100% (PO = IV linezolid)	20 mcg/mL
CAP							
Typical CAP	Streptococcus pneumoniae Haemophilus influenzae Moraxella catarrhalis	Atypical CAP pathogens Oral anaerobes[c]	Doxycycline[b]	100 mg (PO) q12h	1–2 wk	93% (PO = IV doxycycline)	4 mcg/mL
			Levofloxacin	500 mg (PO) q24h		99% (PO = IV levofloxacin)	8 mcg/mL
			Moxifloxacin	400 mg (PO) q24h		90% (PO = IV moxifloxacin)	4.5 mcg/mL
Atypical CAP	Mycoplasma pneumoniae Legionnaire disease	Typical CAP pathogens	Doxycycline[b]	100 mg (PO) q12h	2–3 wk	93% (PO = IV doxycycline)	4 mcg/mL
			Levofloxacin	500 mg (PO) q24h		99% (PO = IV levofloxacin)	8 mcg/mL
			Moxifloxacin	400 mg (PO) q24h		90% (PO = IV moxifloxacin)	4.5 mcg/mL

(continued on next page)

Table 4
(continued)

Clinical Syndromes	Usual Pathogens	Nonpathogens in This Setting	Optimal Oral Therapy	Usual Dosage[a]	Usual Duration	Percent Orally Absorbed	Peak Serum Level
UTIs							
Cystitis	GNB	CoNS MSSA MRSA VSE VRE	Amoxicillin	1 g (PO) q8h	1 wk	90% (PO = IV ampicillin)	14 mcg/mL (urine level = 1000 mcg/mL)
			Nitrofurantoin	100 mg (PO) q12h	1–3 d	80% (PO)	1 mg/mL (urine level = 100 mg/mL)
			TMP-SMX	1 SS tablet (PO) q6h		98% (PO = TMP-SMX)	8 mcg/mL urine levels = 60 mcg (TMP)/150 mcg (SMX)
	VSE	VRE GNB	Amoxicillin	1 g (PO) q8h	1 wk	90% (PO = IV)	14 mcg/mL (urine level = 1000 mcg/mL)
			Nitrofurantoin	100 mg (PO) q12h		80% (PO = IV ampicillin or levofloxacin)	1 mg/mL (urine level = 100 mg/mL)
	VRE	VSE GNB	Nitrofurantoin	100 mg (PO) q12h	1 wk	80% (PO = IV ampicillin or levofloxacin)	1 mg/mL (urine level = 100 mg/mL)
			Linezolid	600 mg (PO) q12h		100% (PO = IV linezolid)	20 mcg/mL
	MDR GNB	CoNS VSE VRE MSSA MRSA	Nitrofurantoin	100 mg (PO) q12h	1 wk	80% (PO = IV ampicillin or levofloxacin)	1 mg/mL (urine level = 100 mcg/mL)
			Doxycycline	200 mg (PO) q12h		93% (PO = IV doxycycline)	8 mcg/mL (urine levels = >300 mcg/mL)
			Fosfomycin	3 g (PO) × 72 h × 2		37% (PO = IV fosfomycin)	26 mg/mL (urine level = 1000 mcg/mL)

Abbreviations: CoNS, coagulase negative staphylococci; GNB, gram-negative bacilli; VRE, vancomycin resistant enterococci; VSE, vancomycin sensitive enterococci.
[a] Usual adult dosage with normal renal function.
[b] Begin therapy with a loading dose of 200 mg.
[c] All CAP antibiotic selections are also active against the oral anaerobes causing aspiration pneumonia.

azithromycin. However, if one uses doxycycline or a "respiratory quinolone" (levofloxacin or moxifloxacin) both typical and atypical coverage is provided with one antibiotic.[2,12–15]

In cystitis, the clinician must verify the diagnosis and verify the bacteriuria is accompanied by substantial pyuria. Antibiotics concentration at the infection site works in favor of the physician with cystitis because most antibiotics achieve high concentration in urine. Urinary antibiotic concentrations are useful in overcoming relative resistance of some uropathogens; for example, oral penicillin can easily eradicate resistant (not multidrug resistant [MDR]) *Escherichia coli* from the urine. Interpretation of susceptibilities of uropathogens should take high urinary concentration into account.

As a general rule, if a uropathogen is reported to be susceptible, it likely is. However, if reported as resistant, the resistance may be relative resistance easily overcome by high urinary levels. The antibiotics suggested in taking these factors into account to provide guidance for physicians[2,23] (**Table 4**).

In summary, oral antibiotic therapy for most infectious diseases, but particularly SSTIs, CAP, and cystitis, provide great advantages for the patient health care system and makes good ASP sense.

REFERENCES

1. Cunha CB. Principles of antimicrobial stewardship. In: LaPlante KL, Cunha CB, Morrill HJ, et al, editors. Antimicrobial stewardship: principles and practice. London: CABI Press; 2017. p. 1–8.
2. Cunha CB, Cunha BA, editors. Antibiotic essentials. 15th edition. New Delhi (India): Jay Pee Med Publishers; 2017.
3. Sensakovic JE, Smith LG. Oral antibiotic treatment of infectious diseases. Med Clin North Am 2001;85:115–23.
4. Cunha BA. Intravenous to oral antibiotic switch therapy. Drugs Today (BARC) 2001;37:311–9.
5. Cunha BA. Oral antibiotic therapy of serious systematic infections. Med Clin North Am 2006;90:1197–222.
6. Quintiliani R, Nightingale CH. Transitional antibiotic therapy. Infect Dis Clin Pract 1994;3(Suppl):161–7.
7. Nightingale CH, Grant EM, Quintiliani R. Pharmacodynamics and pharmacokinetics of levofloxacin. Chemotherapy 2000;46:6–14.
8. Siegel RE, Halpern NA, Almenoff PL, et al. A prospective randomized study of inpatient intravenous antibiotics for community-acquired pneumonia: the optimal duration of therapy. Chest 1996;110:963–71.
9. Altemeier WA, Culbertson WR, Coith RI. The intestinal absorption of oral antibiotics in traumatic shock: an experimental study. Surg Gynecol Obstet 1951;92:707–11.
10. Power BM, Forbes AM, van Heerden PV, et al. Pharmacokinetics of drugs used in critically ill adults. Clin Pharmacokinet 1998;34:25–56.
11. Rebuck JA, Fish DN, Abraham E. Pharmacokinetics of intravenous and oral levofloxacin in critically ill adults in a medical intensive care unit. Pharmacotherapy 2002;22:1216–25.
12. Cunha BA. Oral or intravenous-to-oral antibiotic switch therapy for treating patients with community acquired pneumonia. Am J Med 2001;111:412–3.
13. Ramirez JA, Bordon J. Early switch from intravenous to oral antibiotics in hospitalized patients with bacteremic community acquired Streptococcus pneumoniae pneumonia. Arch Intern Med 2001;161:848–50.

14. Cunha BA. Doxycycline for community acquired pneumonia. Clin Infect Dis 2003; 37:870.
15. Torres A, Muir JF, Corris P, et al. Effectiveness of oral moxifloxacin in standard first line therapy in community acquired pneumonia in community acquired pneumonia. Eur Respir J 2003;21:135–43.
16. Cunha BA. Oral antibiotics to treat MRSA infections. J Hosp Infect 2005;60: 88–90.
17. Cunha BA. Empiric therapy of community-acquired pneumonia: guidelines for the perplexed? Chest 2004;125:1913–9.
18. Cunha BA. Empiric oral monotherapy for hospitalized patients with community acquired pneumonia: an idea whose time has come. Eur J Clin Microbiol Infect Dis 2004;23:78–81.
19. Hoelken G, Talan D, Larsen LS, et al. Efficacy and safety of sequential moxifloxacin for treatment of community-acquired pneumonia associated with atypical pathogens. Eur J Clin Microbiol Infect Dis 2004;23:772–5.
20. Cunha BA. Minocycline versus doxycycline for methicillin-resistant Staphylococcus aureus (MRSA): in vitro susceptibility versus in vivo effectiveness. Int J Antimicrob Agents 2010;35:517–8.
21. Cunha BA, Baron J, Cunha CB. Similarities and differences between doxycycline and minocycline: clinical and antimicrobial stewardship considerations. Eur J Clin Microbiol Infect Dis 2018;37:15–20.
22. Marrie TJ, Lau CY, Wheeler SL, et al. A controlled trial of critical pathway for treatment of community-acquired pneumonia. CAPITAL study investigators. Community-acquired pneumonia intervention trial assessing levofloxacin. JAMA 2000;283:749–55.
23. Kucers A, Crowe SM, Grayson MI, et al, editors. The use of antibiotics. 5th edition. Oxford (England): Butterworth-Heinemann; 1977.
24. Bryskier A, editor. Antimicrobial agents. Washington, DC: ASM Press; 2005.
25. Cunha BA. Minocycline, often forgotten, but preferred to trimethoprim-sulfamethoxazole or doxycycline for the treatment of community acquired methicillin-resistant Staphylococcus aureus skin and soft tissue infections. Int J Antimicrob Agents 2013;42:497–9.

Role of Technology in Antimicrobial Stewardship

Derek N. Bremmer, PharmD[a],*, Tamara L. Trienski, PharmD[a],
Thomas L. Walsh, MD[b], Matthew A. Moffa, DO[b]

KEYWORDS

- Antimicrobial stewardship • Electronic medical record • Social media • Technology

KEY POINTS

- Incorporating the electronic medical record and clinical decision support systems to perform antimicrobial stewardship activities is an important avenue for time optimization.
- Web sites and mobile applications are able to provide vast amounts of medical information that is easily retrievable.
- With the increase in pertinent information available regarding antimicrobial utilization, social media can be used to disseminate up-to-date educational materials to providers and patients.

INTRODUCTION

Because of the increasing plague of antimicrobial resistance (AR) and antibiotic misuse, antimicrobial stewardship programs (ASPs) are now a mandatory entity in all US hospitals.[1,2] Depending on the resources available to the institution, ASPs can target low-hanging fruit, such as intravenous (IV) to oral conversions, or high-impact targets, such as blood culture automated reviews with prospective audit and feedback.[3,4] The more an ASP attempts to take on, the more important time efficiency becomes. Technological advances, such as the electronic medical record (EMR), clinical decision support systems (CDSS), mobile applications (apps), and social media, are important avenues for ASPs to optimize their time.[5]

INCORPORATING THE ELECTRONIC MEDICAL RECORD

By simply implementing an EMR, Cook and colleagues[5] showed that an ASP can increase the number of charts reviewed and interventions made compared with paper

Disclosure Statement: The authors have no potential conflicts of interest to disclose in the commercial or private sectors.
[a] Department of Pharmacy, Allegheny General Hospital, Allegheny Health Network, 320 East North Avenue, Pittsburgh, PA 15212, USA; [b] Division of Infectious Diseases, Allegheny General Hospital, Allegheny Health Network, 320 East North Avenue, 4th Floor East Wing, Suite 406, Pittsburgh, PA 15212, USA
* Corresponding author.
E-mail address: Derek.Bremmer@ahn.org

Med Clin N Am 102 (2018) 955–963
https://doi.org/10.1016/j.mcna.2018.05.007
0025-7125/18/© 2018 Elsevier Inc. All rights reserved.

medical.theclinics.com

charts, which correlated with a 28.8% decrease in broad-spectrum antimicrobial use (AU). The antimicrobial stewardship capabilities of 2 of the most common EMRs, Epic and PowerChart [Cerner], have recently been reviewed.[6,7] Some of the capabilities include tracking interventions, dose checking alerts, best practice alerts, antimicrobial time-outs, restriction processes, and IV to oral monitoring. All of these are key components to a successful ASP.

One of the most common ways to use the EMR for antimicrobial stewardship is to incorporate antibiotic restriction processes.[6,8] Using the order entry system (Siemens/Cerner Invision), Lambl and colleagues[8] placed a restriction to fire whenever a fluoroquinolone or clindamycin was prescribed. This restriction prompted the provider with a rationale for avoiding these agents and a list of approved indications. If a clinician selected a nonapproved indication, a phone intervention was triggered for review by a pharmacist or infectious diseases (ID) specialist. This built-in restriction resulted in a 91% reduction in days of therapy per 1000 patient days for clindamycin and fluoroquinolones, which in turn correlated with a 24% reduction in hospital-acquired *Clostridium difficile* infections ($P = .05$).

Another tactic is to implement an antibiotic time-out into the EMR. In one study, the impact of an antibiotic time-out was compared with the previous workflow, which involved vancomycin and piperacillin/tazobactam use beyond 3 days requiring approval by the ID fellow, pharmacist, or attending physician. With the time-out, the ID approval was waived and antibiotic continuation was approved if the provider completed a renewal template. The electronic antibiotic time-out led to similar rates of antibiotic discontinuation compared with the historical requirement for approval from an ID practitioner but was much less labor intensive.[9] Another study used a daily prompt in the EMR that reminded clinicians to ensure all antimicrobials have an appropriate indication and stop/review date recorded. On implementation of this intervention, 96% of orders were recorded to have an indication and stop date.[10]

When antimicrobial stewardship interventions are integrated into the EMR, it is important to keep in mind the needs of the hospital practitioners. An overabundance of alerts can cause alert fatigue with eventual desensitization. It is also important to keep the workflow efficient and allow deviations from the typical order set to prevent loss of autonomy.[11] Structuring interventions to the sociocultural antibiotic prescribing practices and technologically available resources is critical.

CLINICAL DECISION SUPPORT SYSTEMS

Electronic CDSSs, whether contained within an EMR (eg, Epic's Antimicrobial Stewardship Module) or a stand-alone product (eg, Theradoc [Premier], Sentri7 [Wolters Kluwer]), can play a critical role in ASPs. CDSSs have the ability to generate real-time alerts and reports to help ASPs identify patients for potential interventions.

Real-time alerts can include the following:

- Patients with positive blood cultures
- Patients with rapid diagnostic test results
- Patients ordered a specified antimicrobial
- Patients with cultures for a specified microorganism (eg, *Staphylococcus aureus* or *Pseudomonas aeruginosa*)

Reports can include the following:

- Patients on antimicrobials for defined time periods
- Patients who are candidates for IV to oral conversion
- Patients with decreased renal function

- Patients with a potential drug-bug mismatch who might be on inappropriate therapy

Several studies have demonstrated that CDSSs increase the number of antimicrobial interventions that can be made. Huber and colleagues,[12] at a small community hospital, showed that implementation of Sentri7 provided an 87% increase in the number of antibiotic-related interventions (144 vs 270 interventions in the 3-month preimplementation and 3-month postimplementation periods, respectively). After implementation of TheraDoc at a large academic medical center, Ghamrawi and colleagues[13] demonstrated a significant time reduction in both de-escalation and escalation to appropriate antimicrobial therapy.

Another area where CDSSs can be a major asset is in the electronic reporting of AU and AR data to the Centers for Disease Control and Prevention's National Healthcare Safety Network (NHSN). Currently this is voluntary, but the NHSN AU and/or AR reporting has been identified as one option for eligible hospitals to meet the Public Health Registry reporting under stage 3 of the Centers for Medicare and Medicaid Services' Meaningful Use Program.[14] This information must be submitted electronically in Health Level Clinical Document Architecture format. Manual data entry is not available for the Antimicrobial Use and Resistance (AUR) Module.[15] **Table 1** provides a list of AUR vendors and their data transmission capabilities.[16]

Despite the substantial advantages of CDSSs for ASPs, there are disadvantages or limitations of which to be aware. Disadvantages of CDSSs center around cost and information technology (IT) support. Initial and yearly subscription fees of CDSSs can be costly to an institution, ranging from $100,000 to $500,000 annually.[7] Additionally, extensive IT support is needed for the development and implementation of CDSSs, especially when integrated in an EMR. Although the costs may be substantial, CDSSs have clearly shown their role in optimizing antimicrobial utilization and have shown to be cost-effective.[17]

Table 1
CDC's National Healthcare Safety Network (NHSN) Antimicrobial Use (AU) and Antimicrobial Resistance (AR) module reporting vendors

Vendor Name	AU Reporting	AR Reporting
Asolva, Inc.	Yes	
Atlas Development Corporation		
Bluebird IMS, Inc.	Yes	Yes
Cerner	Yes	Yes
Epic Systems Corporation	Yes	Yes
Baxter Healthcare/ICNet	Yes	
Ilum Health Solutions	Yes	
Lumed with bioMerieux, Inc.		
MedMined™ services from BD	Yes	Yes
Midas Healthy Analytics Solutions – Conduent		
RL Solutions	Yes	
Sentri7 by Wolters Kluwer	Yes	
TheraDoc – Premier	Yes	Yes
QC Pathfinder – Venca Technologies		
VigiLanz Corporation	Yes	Yes

Adapted from Society of Infectious Diseases Pharmacists (SIDP). AUR vendors. Available at: https://www.sidp.org/resources/Documents/AUR%20List/sidp-aur-vendors%2010-20-17.pdf. Accessed June 1, 2018; with permission.

MOBILE APPLICATIONS

With the ubiquitous nature of smartphones, information is now literally at our fingertips. Web sites and mobile apps are able to provide vast amounts of medical information that is easily retrievable in a matter of seconds. A 2014 survey by Epocrates, one of the most downloaded medical apps, found that 80% of clinicians use their mobile devices in their professional workflow.[18] Mobile devices have been shown to improve clinical decision-making and allow health professionals to be more efficient in their work practices.[19] Incorporating this technology to improve antimicrobial stewardship efforts is a rather new strategy with unbound potential.

Finding relevant and reliable ID apps can be difficult. In a 2013 review, more than 1200 ID apps were identified from the Apple and Google Play app stores. However, only 24 were found to be relevant, easy to navigate, written in English, and developed by trustworthy sources.[20] Developing institutional ID apps may be a more effective format for antimicrobial prescribing guidance. Traditionally, physicians are issued printed pocket guides for antimicrobial prescribing. In a British study, paper-based pocket guides were replaced with a smartphone app. The app was used significantly more than the pocket guide and led users to more frequently challenge inappropriate prescribing by their colleagues, and users were more aware of the importance of antimicrobial stewardship.[21] In another study that converted antimicrobial prescribing policy to a mobile app, a significant increase in compliance with policy was seen in the specialty of surgery.[22] In an observational before/after study in Brazil, an institutional app consisting of a guidance manual for the choice of antimicrobials according to the site of infection was implemented. The app was linked with laboratory culture results and a susceptibility profile, allowing a real-time update. The monthly average consumption of piperacillin/tazobactam and meropenem was significantly decreased after the app implementation, whereas the consumption of aminoglycosides and cefepime significantly increased. The susceptibility profiles of meropenem and polymyxin improved, and there was a net savings of nearly $300,000 during the 12 months after app implementation.[23] Institutional apps have also been developed to assist with inpatient penicillin allergies. At Massachusetts General Hospital, the implementation of a computerized guideline application with clinical decision support significantly increased penicillin or cephalosporin use nearly 2-fold in patients previously labeled with a penicillin allergy.[24]

Although most antimicrobial stewardship mobile app efforts have been confined to the inpatient acute care setting and geared toward health care professionals, there is the potential for electronic resources to educate both medical trainees and the public regarding AU and resistance. Integrating smartphone apps in antimicrobial stewardship curricula was found to significantly increase antibiogram use and improved syndrome prescription among second-year medical students.[25] In a 2016 review of the Apple and Google Play app stores, very few apps (including games) targeting antimicrobial prescribing/stewardship/resistance were found that were geared toward the public.[26] In a cross-sectional study surveying 99 patients, 66%, 50%, and 100% wanted information on the cause of their infection, optimal management of the infection, and antimicrobial-specific information, respectively. About half of the respondents supported doctors using electronic platforms to access medical information during a consultation. These findings suggest that there is a gap and demand by patients for an app that provides antimicrobial- and infection-specific information.[27]

SOCIAL MEDIA

Clinical practice guidelines are published with increasing regularity to ensure high-quality, evidence-based care. Although physicians typically agree with national guidelines, the lack of accompanying tactics for local implementation is an arduous obstacle.[28] Despite their availability, guidelines for antimicrobial prescribing are not consistently followed by clinicians.[29–32] ASPs can facilitate multidisciplinary development of institution-specific, evidence-based practice guidelines that incorporate local microbiology and resistance patterns.[30–32] However, it remains difficult to get primary providers to use these clinical tools. ASPs must be able to disseminate these educational materials to the primary prescribers of antimicrobials to effectively and efficiently optimize antimicrobial prescribing.[33]

Historically, new information is obtained via utilization of medical journals, educational conferences, and other didactic sessions.[34] Alternative techniques for clinician education regarding antimicrobial therapy are needed to supplement traditional educational methods. Social media, including Twitter, Facebook, and Instagram, have demonstrated success in education and consumer advertising.[35] As these social media platforms exist to bring attention to issues, using them to help educate clinicians about appropriate utilization of antimicrobials seems a natural fit.[36] Via the use of social media, clinicians are able to deliver easily accessible, real-time, high-yield information to peers, colleagues, trainees, and non–health care professionals (HCPs). Social media is being used for education of nursing and medical students and for continuing education for other HCPs.[37,38] A survey among physicians who were active participants in social media was conducted to determine the perceived benefits and challenges of using social media. The main reasons for social media use were to connect with colleagues, networking with a world-wide community, sharing of knowledge, branding, and engaging in continuing medical education.[39]

Twitter is a free social networking service that was founded in 2006. It is the 13th most visited Web site worldwide and has more than 300 million monthly visitors who send more than 58 million tweets per day.[34,40,41] Twitter has proven useful as a learning tool in educational settings where the use of this platform in college courses helped enhance communication with faculty, increased student engagement, and improved course grades.[42,43] Twitter is also emerging as a valuable platform for HCPs, as more than 75,000 HCPs send more than 150,000 tweets per day, with nearly a third of these from the United States.[34] In a survey conducted by Panahi and colleagues,[39] physicians cited limited time to read primary journal articles due to busy schedules. Twitter was able to keep them current in regard to updates in their field, as they were able to quickly review peer-reviewed information. In the first 12 months after creation of the International Urology Journal Club, this online Twitter journal club had 189 active participants from 19 countries. They were able to exceed the reach of most traditional journal clubs by tweeting an average of 195 tweets monthly, while generating a reach of 130,832 per month.[44] Additionally, Twitter can dramatically grow the available audience for academic conferences.[45] Indeed, urologists used Twitter to augment the content of the European Association of Urology meeting, as 5903 tweets reached more than 7 million users.[46]

Facebook is a for-profit corporation and an online social media/social networking service that was launched in 2004. Eighty-three percent of Facebook users are between 18 and 29 years old, which comprises most medical students and house staff.[47] Pisano and colleagues[33] performed a quasi-experimental study aimed at improving internal medicine residents' knowledge of appropriate antibiotic use as well as increasing the utilization of local order sets and clinical decision-making pathways through the use of social media. Fifty-five residents were enrolled and asked to follow the institution's ASP on Facebook and/or Twitter for a 6-month period. Social media was used to promote the institution's ASP Web site, pathways, and order sets. Questions about antibiotic prescribing were posted and tweeted, and subsequent answers were revealed the following day. Tests and surveys administered before and after the intervention showed that the enrolled residents improved their knowledge of antimicrobial prescribing. Additionally, they were more aware of how to access the ASP Web site and clinical pathways. The percent of residents who self-reported using the clinical pathways increased from 33% to 61%.

With the increase in new, pertinent information available regarding antimicrobial utilization and ever-changing guidelines (both nationally and locally), multiple new modalities for education can be used to supplement traditional educational methods. Social media can be used to disseminate up-to-date educational materials, which are likely to appeal to younger generations that rely heavily on social media. Social media has the capability to highlight and propagate information regarding antimicrobial utilization by reaching HCPs in a widespread and timely manner. By leveraging these platforms, ASPs may be better equipped to adjust to the constantly evolving technologic landscape and educational needs of their target audiences.

SUMMARY

Using the EMR and CDSSs are core components of a successful ASP. These technologies allow an ASP to impact a larger patient population with more efficiency. Apps and social media have the capability to highlight and propagate educational information in a widespread and timely manner. Applying these resources can greatly enhance antimicrobial education to patients and HCPs.

REFERENCES

1. Boucher HW, Talbot GH, Bradley JS, et al. Bad bugs, no drugs: no ESKAPE! An update from the Infectious Diseases Society of America. Clin Infect Dis 2009; 48(1):1–12.
2. The Joint Commission on Hospital Accreditation. APPROVED: new antimicrobial stewardship standard. Jt Comm Perspect 2016;36(7):1, 3–4, 8.
3. Goff DA, Bauer KA, Reed EE, et al. Is the "low-hanging fruit" worth picking for antimicrobial stewardship programs? Clin Infect Dis 2012;55(4):587–92.
4. Wenzler E, Wang F, Goff DA, et al. An automated, pharmacist-driven initiative improves quality of care for staphylococcus aureus bacteremia. Clin Infect Dis 2017;65(2):194–200.
5. Cook PP, Rizzo S, Gooch M, et al. Sustained reduction in antimicrobial use and decrease in methicillin-resistant Staphylococcus aureus and Clostridium difficile infections following implementation of an electronic medical record at a tertiary-care teaching hospital. J Antimicrob Chemother 2011;66(1): 205–9.
6. Pogue JM, Potoski BA, Postelnick M, et al. Bringing the "power" to Cerner's PowerChart for antimicrobial stewardship. Clin Infect Dis 2014;59(3):416–24.
7. Kullar R, Goff DA, Schulz LT, et al. The "epic" challenge of optimizing antimicrobial stewardship: the role of electronic medical records and technology. Clin Infect Dis 2013;57(7):1005–13.
8. Lambl BB, Kaufman N, Kurowski J, et al. Does electronic stewardship work? J Am Med Inform Assoc 2017;24(5):981–5.
9. Graber CJ, Jones MM, Glassman PA, et al. Taking an antibiotic time-out: utilization and usability of a self-stewardship time-out program for renewal of vancomycin and piperacillin-tazobactam. Hosp Pharm 2015;50(11):1011–24.

10. Allan PA, Newman MJ, Oehmen R, et al. The use of daily electronic prompts to help improve antimicrobial stewardship in a critical care unit. J Infect Prev 2016;17(4):179–84.
11. Chung P, Scandlyn J, Dayan PS, et al. Working at the intersection of context, culture, and technology: provider perspectives on antimicrobial stewardship in the emergency department using electronic health record clinical decision support. Am J Infect Control 2017;45(11):1198–202.
12. Huber SR, Fullas F, Nelson KR, et al. Retrospective evaluation of pharmacist interventions on use of antimicrobials using a clinical surveillance software in a small community hospital. Pharmacy (Basel) 2016;4(4) [pii:E32].
13. Ghamrawi RJ, Kantorovich A, Bauer SR, et al. Evaluation of antimicrobial stewardship-related alerts using a clinical decision support system. Hosp Pharm 2017;52(10):679–84.
14. Centers for Disease Control and Prevention (CDC). Using NHSN AUR Module for Meaningful Use stage 3. Available at: https://www.cdc.gov/nhsn/pdfs/cda/mu3-facility-guidance.pdf. Accessed January 19, 2018.
15. Centers for Disease Control and Prevention (CDC). Antimicrobial Use and Resistance (AUR) Module. 2018; Available at: https://www.cdc.gov/nhsn/PDFs/pscManual/11pscAURcurrent.pdf.Accessed January 19, 2018.
16. Society of Infectious Diseases Pharmacists (SIDP). AUR vendors. Available at: https://www.sidp.org/resources/Documents/AUR%20List/sidp-aur-vendors%2010-20-17.pdf. Accessed June 1, 2018.
17. Calloway S, Akilo HA, Bierman K. Impact of a clinical decision support system on pharmacy clinical interventions, documentation efforts, and costs. Hosp Pharm 2013;48(9):744–52.
18. Epocrates. Mobile trends report overview. 2014. Available at: http://www.epocrates.com/sites/default/files/MT14_WP_03.pdf. Accessed November 28, 2017.
19. Mickan S, Tilson JK, Atherton H, et al. Evidence of effectiveness of health care professionals using handheld computers: a scoping review of systematic reviews. J Med Internet Res 2013;15(10):e212.
20. Moodley A, Mangino JE, Goff DA. Review of infectious diseases applications for iPhone/iPad and Android: from pocket to patient. Clin Infect Dis 2013;57(8):1145–54.
21. Panesar P, Jones A, Aldous A, et al. Attitudes and behaviours to antimicrobial prescribing following introduction of a smartphone app. PLoS One 2016;11(4):e0154202.
22. Charani E, Gharbi M, Moore LSP, et al. Effect of adding a mobile health intervention to a multimodal antimicrobial stewardship programme across three teaching hospitals: an interrupted time series study. J Antimicrob Chemother 2017;72(6):1825–31.
23. Tuon FF, Gasparetto J, Wollmann LC, et al. Mobile health application to assist doctors in antibiotic prescription - an approach for antibiotic stewardship. Braz J Infect Dis 2017;21(6):660–4.
24. Blumenthal KG, Wickner PG, Hurwitz S, et al. Tackling inpatient penicillin allergies: assessing tools for antimicrobial stewardship. J Allergy Clin Immunol 2017;140(1):154–61.e6.
25. Nori P, Madaline T, Munjal I, et al. Developing interactive antimicrobial stewardship and infection prevention curricula for diverse learners: a tailored approach. Open Forum Infect Dis 2017;4(3):ofx117.

26. Micallef C, Kildonavaciute K, Castro-Sanchez E, et al. Is there a role for a bespoke app on antimicrobial stewardship targeting patients and the public? Clin Infect Dis 2016;63(1):140–1.

27. Micallef C, McLeod M, Castro-Sanchez E, et al. An evidence-based antimicrobial stewardship smartphone app for hospital outpatients: survey-based needs assessment among patients. JMIR Mhealth Uhealth 2016;4(3):e83.

28. Lomas J, Anderson GM, Domnick-Pierre K, et al. Do practice guidelines guide practice? The effect of a consensus statement on the practice of physicians. N Engl J Med 1989;321(19):1306–11.

29. Walsh TL, DiSilvio BE, Speredelozzi D, et al. Evaluation of management of uncomplicated community-acquired pneumonia: a retrospective assessment. Infect Dis Clin Pract (Baltim Md) 2017;25(2):71–5.

30. Walsh TL, Bremmer DN, Moffa MA, et al. Effect of antimicrobial stewardship program guidance on the management of uncomplicated skin and soft tissue infections in hospitalized adults. Mayo Clinic Proceedings: Innovations, Quality & Outcomes 2017;1(1):91–9.

31. Jenkins TC, Knepper BC, Sabel AL, et al. Decreased antibiotic utilization after implementation of a guideline for inpatient cellulitis and cutaneous abscess. Arch Intern Med 2011;171(12):1072–9.

32. Avdic E, Cushinotto LA, Hughes AH, et al. Impact of an antimicrobial stewardship intervention on shortening the duration of therapy for community-acquired pneumonia. Clin Infect Dis 2012;54(11):1581–7.

33. Pisano J, Pettit N, Bartlett A, et al. Social media as a tool for antimicrobial stewardship. Am J Infect Control 2016;44(11):1231–6.

34. Goff DA, Kullar R, Newland JG. Review of twitter for infectious diseases clinicians: useful or a waste of time? Clin Infect Dis 2015;60(10):1533–40.

35. Galiatsatos P, Porto-Carreiro F, Hayashi J, et al. The use of social media to supplement resident medical education - the SMART-ME initiative. Med Educ Online 2016;21(1):29332.

36. Conway LJ, Knighton SC. Journal club: social media as an antimicrobial stewardship tool. Am J Infect Control 2017;45(3):293–4.

37. Cartledge P, Miller M, Phillips B. The use of social-networking sites in medical education. Med Teach 2013;35(10):847–57.

38. Schmitt TL, Sims-Giddens SS, Booth RG. Social media use in nursing education. Online J Issues Nurs 2012;17(3):2.

39. Panahi S, Watson J, Partridge H. Social media and physicians: exploring the benefits and challenges. Health Informatics J 2016;22(2):99–112.

40. Wikipedia. Twitter, Inc. Available at: https://en.wikipedia.org/wiki/Twitter. Accessed January 12, 2017.

41. Statista. Most famous social network sites worldwide as of September 2017, ranked by number of active users (in millions). Available at: https://www.statista.com/statistics/272014/global-social-networks-ranked-by-number-of-users/. Accessed January 12, 2017.

42. Junco R, Heiberger G, Loken E. The effect of Twitter on college student engagement and grades. J Comput Assist Learn 2011;27(2):119–32.

43. Junco R, Elavsky CM, Heiberger G. Putting twitter to the test: assessing outcomes for student collaboration, engagement and success. Br J Educ Technol 2013;44(2):273–87.

44. Thangasamy IA, Leveridge M, Davies BJ, et al. international urology journal club via twitter: 12-month experience. Eur Urol 2014;66(1):112–7.

45. Cochran A, Kao LS, Gusani NJ, et al. Use of twitter to document the 2013 academic surgical congress. J Surg Res 2014;190(1):36–40.
46. Wilkinson SE, Basto MY, Perovic G, et al. The social media revolution is changing the conference experience: analytics and trends from eight international meetings. BJU Int 2015;115(5):839–46.
47. Rainie L, Brenner J, Purcell K. Photos and videos as social currency online. Washington, DC: Pew Research Center; 2012. Available at: http://www.pewinternet.org/2012/09/13/photos-and-videos-as-social-currency-online/. Accessed January 12, 2017.

Metrics of Antimicrobial Stewardship Programs

Amy L. Brotherton, PharmD

KEYWORDS

• Antimicrobial stewardship • Antibiotic use • Stewardship metrics • Benchmarking

KEY POINTS

- Appropriate metrics are necessary to measure the quality, clinical, and financial impacts of antimicrobial stewardship programs.
- Antimicrobial stewardship metrics are categorized into antibiotic use measures, process measures, quality measures, costs, and clinical outcome measures.
- Traditionally, antimicrobial stewardship metrics have focused on antibiotic use, antibiotic costs, and process measures.
- With health care reform, practice should shift to focusing on the clinical impact of stewardship programs over financial impact.
- More research is needed to define optimal clinical outcome measures; these metrics should be further developed, standardized, and validated for internal and external benchmarking purposes.
- Outpatient antimicrobial stewardship is a novel area and requires metrics for adequate program evaluation; more research is needed to determine optimal metrics in this setting.

INTRODUCTION

The Infectious Diseases Society of America/Society of Healthcare Epidemiology of America (IDSA/SHEA) Antimicrobial Stewardship (AMS) guidelines and the Centers for Disease Control and Prevention (CDC) Core Elements of Hospital Antibiotic Stewardship Programs (ASP) promote ASPs to enhance patient care by improving appropriate use of antimicrobial therapy, decreasing collateral damage, and improving patient outcomes.[1,2] Traditionally, ASP metrics have centered on "low-hanging fruit," including antimicrobial consumption, antimicrobial costs, and process measures.[3–7] Guidance exists regarding the most important metrics for antimicrobial use and costs[1,2]; but few metrics for measuring quality of antimicrobial use and clinical outcomes have been validated and incorporated into routine program assessments.[8,9]

Funding Support: The author has nothing to disclose.
Conflicts of Interest: The author has nothing to disclose.
Infectious Diseases, Department of Pharmacy, The Miriam Hospital, 164 Summit Avenue, Providence, RI 02906, USA
E-mail address: amy.brotherton@lifespan.org

With health care reform and the shift from fee-for-service models to quality of care, ASP programs should refocus their energy on higher-level outcomes metrics.[10] Limitations to proposed outcomes metrics include the presence of confounding factors; difficulty in attributing an improvement in outcomes directly to an ASP intervention; and the feasibility of extracting metrics, performing meaningful analyses, and translating results into actionable conclusions.[6,8,10] **Table 1** provides an introduction to potential useful inpatient ASP metrics based on recommendations from the IDSA/SHEA ASP Guidelines and the CDC's Core Elements for Hospital ASP. Although ASP initiatives have historically concentrated on the inpatient setting, the importance of

Table 1
IDSA/SHEA ASP recommendations and CDC's core elements of ASP: potential metrics to consider

Recommendation	Potential Associated Metric(s)
Develop facility-specific clinical practice guidelines for infectious diseases syndromes[2]	• Compliance with guidelines • Clinical outcomes related to the specific infectious disease syndrome
Implement interventions designed to reduce use of antibiotics associated with high risk of CDI[2]	• Use of high-risk antibiotics associated with CDI • Incidence of CDI • Incidence of CDI related to antimicrobial therapy
Implement interventions to increase appropriate use of oral antibiotics for initial therapy and timely transition from IV to PO antibiotics[2]	• Compliance with IV to PO interventions • Use of IV therapy when PO was appropriate • Adverse effects of IV vs PO therapy • Length of hospitalization in relationship to IV vs PO therapy
Implement guidelines and strategies to reduce antibiotic therapy to the shortest effective duration[2]	• Compliance with recommended duration of therapy as stated in guidelines • Duration of therapy • DOT
Use rapid viral testing for respiratory pathogens to reduce the use of inappropriate antibiotics[2]	• Compliance with recommendation to stop antibiotics in setting of viral illness • Number of patients with viral illness receiving unnecessary antibiotics
Monitor antibiotic use as measured by DOT in preference to DDD[2]	• DOT/1000 patient days • DOT/1000 days present
Measure antibiotic costs based on prescriptions or administrations instead of purchasing data[2]	• Antimicrobial costs (based on prescriptions or administrations)
Monitor process measures[1]	• Documentation of treatment indications • Adherence to facility-specific guidelines • Time to initiation or de-escalation of antibiotic therapy • Antibiotic-related adverse events
Monitor antibiotic use[1]	• DOT or DDD/1000 patient days or days present • Measure both overall antibiotic use and focused analyses on specific antibiotics where stewardship interventions are implemented
Monitor outcomes[1]	• Hospital-onset CDI • Antibiotic resistance • Drug cost savings and healthcare savings

Abbreviations: ASP, antimicrobial stewardship program; CDI, *Clostridium difficile* infection; DDD, defined daily dose; DOT, days of therapy; IDSA, Infectious Diseases Society of America; IV, intravenous; PO, oral; SHEA, Society of Healthcare Epidemiology of America.

stewardship throughout the patient care continuum has gained attention as a national priority; thus, establishing outpatient ASP metrics are of equal importance.[11,12] In this article, the various ASP metrics that have been described in the literature, evidence to support these metrics, controversies surrounding metrics, and areas in which future research is necessary are reviewed.

MEASURING ANTIMICROBIAL CONSUMPTION

An underlying goal of any ASP is to curb the unnecessary use of antibiotic therapy. Measuring antimicrobial consumption, stratified by antibiotic, can help identify over-utilization and, thus, is one of the most widely accepted metrics to demonstrate impact for ASPs.[1,2,4,13] Antibiotic use can be further stratified by unit, provider, or service in the hospital to allow for interfacility comparisons. External comparisons to similar institutions can allow for ASP benchmarking on a broader scale.

Historical reporting of antibiotic consumption used simpler methods, such as measuring the proportion of patients who received antimicrobials during hospitalization.[14–16] With current methods, antimicrobial consumption is expressed as a rate, with the numerator as the consumption metric and the denominator as a measurement of person time at risk for antimicrobial exposure (ie, hospital census). The 2 "numerators" most commonly used include the defined daily dose (DDD) and days of therapy (DOT).[2,17] The 2 "denominators" most commonly used include patient days and days present.[18] The differences between these methods are reviewed as follows and are described in **Table 2**.

Defined Daily Dose

Traditionally, the chief method for reporting antimicrobial consumption worldwide has been accomplished with the DDD.[13] In the 2007 IDSA/SHEA Guidelines for Developing an Institutional Program to Enhance ASP, DDD was regarded as the recommended metric for measuring antimicrobial use; however, the recently updated guidelines prefer DOT, and DDD is listed as an alternative option.[2,13] The DDD was developed by the World Health Organization (WHO) and remains a gold standard metric for comparing data on drug use between countries outside of the United States where electronic administration data may be unobtainable.[19]

WHO defines the DDD as "the assumed average maintenance dose per day for a drug used for its main indication in adults."[19] It is calculated by determining the aggregate number of grams of antibiotic purchased, dispensed, or administered during a defined period and dividing by the WHO-assigned DDD, an amount in grams used to represent the average daily dose in practice. The result is an estimate of DOT. The WHO Collaborating Center for Drug Statistics Methodology publishes an updated version of the assigned DDDs annually.[19] It is important to note that the WHO-assigned DDD may not always reflect the recommended daily adult dose per package labeling; rather, it may be an average of 2 or more commonly used daily doses (if applicable), with consideration for differences in use in various countries.[19] Additionally, for weight-based dosing, a weight of 70 kg is assumed.[19]

The DDD is commonly used at institutions where administration data cannot be obtained or where it is more feasible to report based on purchasing or dispensing data. Advantages of this metric include ease of calculation and ability to facilitate cost analyses because usage data are reported in grams.[6,17,20] However, there are several disadvantages regarding its accuracy, which is why more recent guideline recommendations favor DOT. Because the metric relies on dose of antibiotic in grams, an underestimation of use could be expected in those with renal insufficiency, which would

Table 2
Antimicrobial consumption metrics

Metric	Definition	Advantages	Disadvantages
Numerator (consumption metric)			
Defined daily dose (DDD)	• Average maintenance dose per day for a drug used for its main indication in adults • Grams of antibiotic administered, purchased, or dispensed divided by WHO-assigned DDD (found on WHO Web site)	• Can be used for international benchmarking as other countries use DDD • Does not require administration data • Facilitates cost analyses	• Discrepancies between WHO-assigned DDD and dose used in practice leads to inaccurate assessment of use • Not appropriate for use in pediatric patients • Not an accurate reflection of use in renal impairment
Days of therapy (DOT)	• Aggregate sum of calendar days during which a patient received any amount of an antibiotic as documented in the eMAR and or BCMA data	• Recommended metric by IDSA/SHEA ASP guidelines • Required for participation in CDCs NHSN AU module (referred to as "antimicrobial days") • Appropriate for use in pediatric patients • Not affected by discrepancies between WHO-assigned DDD and dose used in practice	• Not as useful for international benchmarking as other countries use DDD • Not an accurate reflection of use in renal impairment • Requires administration data, which may not be obtainable in all institutions
Denominator (patient time at risk)			
Patient days	• Manual or electronic count of the number of patients in a location measured at the same time each day (ie, a daily census count at 12 AM)	• Information is readily available from infection control data • Historically the gold standard, ASPs and infection control are familiar with the metric	• May miss a partial patient day on the day of admission or discharge depending on time of daily count • Not used in CDCs NHSN module for reporting AU • Underestimates person time
Days present	• Electronic count of calendar day when a patient is present in a location for any portion of the calendar d based on ADT data	• Used in CDCs NHSN module for reporting AU • Better fit for capturing partial days	• Requires electronic capture of continuous ADT data • overestimates person time especially in units with short stays • Novel metric, ASPs and infection control are less familiar with metric

Abbreviations: ADT, admission-transfer-discharge; AU, antibiotic use; BCMA, bar code medication administration; CDC, Centers for Disease Control and Prevention; eMAR, electronic medication administration record; IDSA, Infectious Diseases Society of America; NHSN, National Healthcare Safety Network; SHEA, Society of Healthcare Epidemiology of America; WHO, World Health Organization.

make for an unfair comparison with an institution or ward with a different census of elderly or renally impaired patients.[6,20,21] Additionally, this metric cannot be used in pediatric patients for whom lower doses and varying weight-based dosing is frequently prescribed.[20] The greatest disadvantage, however, is the risk of discrepancies between the WHO-assigned DDD and the DDD used in current practice, resulting in an inaccurate assessment of antimicrobial use.[6,17,20]

Days of Therapy

DOT is currently the preferred metric for reporting antimicrobial consumption in the United States.[2] It is used by Epic, the leading implementer of electronic medical records in the United States, and the CDC's National Healthcare Safety Network (NHSN) for reporting antimicrobial use.[22,23]

DOT is calculated by tallying the number of calendar days during which a patient received an antibiotic based on administration data, regardless of dose or frequency. Each individual antibiotic received per day is granted 1 DOT; thus, a patient receiving dual antimicrobial therapy for 5 days would be reported as 10 DOTs. This does not necessarily correlate with appropriateness; for example, if a patient were switched from broad-spectrum monotherapy to 2 narrower agents, this would result in increased DOTs.

Like DDD, DOT may underestimate exposure in patients with renal impairment, as it does not account for prolonged dosing intervals or prolonged drug half-lives in the presence of renal dysfunction (ie, when using vancomycin "pulse" dosing). However, it can be used in pediatric patients.[6,20] DOT requires patient-level data, which is both an advantage and a disadvantage, as it inherently improves the accuracy of the metric, but requires electronic medication administration records (eMAR) or bar code medication administration (BCMA) data, which may not be obtainable in every institution.

DDD Versus DOT: Evidence to Date

Discrepancies when comparing DDD versus DOT data have been highlighted in the literature.[17,24,25] Polk and colleagues[17] compared DDD versus DOT results for 130 hospitals and observed poor correlation, often due to dissimilarities between the WHO-assigned DDD and the facility-administered dose. When the daily administered dose was less than the WHO-assigned DDD, such as for piperacillin-tazobactam and ceftriaxone, estimates of use based on DDDs per 1000 patient days were significantly lower than those based on DOTs per 1000 patient days ($P<.001$).[17] For example, for ceftriaxone, the WHO-assigned DDD is listed as 2 g, although a dose of 1 g is often used in the United States, leading to the appearance of "underutilization" when compared with DOT data.[19] The opposite was true when the daily administered dose exceeded the WHO-defined DDD, such as for cefepime and ampicillin-sulbactam.

Alternatively, Dalton and colleagues[26] found only a relatively small difference when comparing the 2 metrics in 32 medical wards in a health system in Canada. However, they did observe a 23% lower DDD when using nursing administration records versus pharmacy dispensing records, indicating that this is another clinically relevant factor to take into consideration when performing antimicrobial use calculations.[26]

The Importance of the Denominator

To make matters more complicated, there are also various denominators used to standardize DOT or DDD for hospital census, the 2 most common being patient days and days present.[18,23] Traditionally, most institutions have used patient days as the person-time denominator.[2,18] Patient days is a manual or electronic count of the number of patients in a given location measured at the same time each day (ie, a daily census count at 12 AM). This information is typically readily available from infection control or administrative data. However, a one-time census count may miss a partial patient day on the day of admission or discharge depending on the time of the daily count.[18]

Days present is a novel method, specifically created for the CDC's NHSN Antibiotic Use (AU) module, and is fit for capturing partial days in hospital locations.[18,23] Days present is an electronic count of patients present in a given location for *any* portion of the calendar day. For example, if a patient were admitted to the hospital on Sunday at 8 PM and discharged on Monday at 8 PM, this would represent 1 patient day based on a 12 AM census count.[18,23] When using days present, however, this would represent 2 days present because the patient was in that specific location at some point during 2 calendar days.

The CDC estimates that days present are roughly 29% higher than patient days for the same month/location.[23] Moehring and colleagues[18] evaluated the difference between using days present versus patient days on antimicrobial use rates and found a similar discrepancy. Using days present as opposed to patient days inflated the denominator by one-third, indicating that antimicrobial consumption rates may appear substantially lower when using days present versus patient days.[18]

There are numerous ways to track and report antimicrobial consumption, none of which are 100% accurate. When making internal or external comparisons, it is important to understand that results may vary significantly depending on both consumption metric used and the metric used for representation of patients at risk. Consistency in metric use over time is important for accurate longitudinal internal and external benchmarking.

National Healthcare Safety Network Antibiotic Use Module and the Standardized Antimicrobial Administration Ratio

The CDC's NHSN has been used for several years for infection control purposes for tracking health care–associated infections. Additionally, an AU module was developed to electronically collect and report monthly DOT data for AMS national benchmarking purposes.[23] The module requires reporting in DOT per 1000 days present based off of administration records only. Reporting is currently voluntary, and facilities must have an information technology infrastructure with the capability of importing data into the module.[8,18,23] A list of self-identified vendors that provide services and software for participation in the module can be found on the Society of Infectious Diseases Pharmacists Web site.[23] Using data reported through the AU module, the CDC has developed an additional metric, the Standardized Antimicrobial Administration Ratio (SAAR).[23,27] The SAAR is calculated by dividing an institution's observed antimicrobial use (ie, DOT) by its predicted or expected antimicrobial use. Expected antimicrobial use is based on predictive modules applied to aggregated national AU data. A statistically significant high SAAR (more than 1) indicates more antimicrobial use than predicted. A statistically significant low SAAR (less than 1) indicates less antimicrobial use than predicted.[23,27] The SAAR is not a definitive measure for inappropriate use; rather, it serves as a starting point for further investigation into use. Over time, this metric could become more valuable as more and more facilities begin participating in the AU module.

QUALITY AND PROCESS MEASURES

Measuring antimicrobial consumption informs use outside of the norm but does not directly measure appropriateness of use. Determining the quality of antimicrobial use (ie, inappropriate vs appropriate use) is an additional task for ASPs and requires patient-level data and further analyses.

The CDC's Core Elements of Hospital ASPs recommend performing periodic assessments to determine quality of antibiotic use.[1] Although there is no one good metric for determining quality in antibiotic prescribing, compliance and/or intervention acceptance rates are appropriate metrics to start with. With every new process, policy, or stewardship intervention, compliance should be measured. When performing daily prospective audit and feedback, physician acceptance or refusal rates should be tracked. These data can be used to identify services or providers that should be targeted for future interventions and educational opportunities. Tracking the amount of time it takes to perform the intervention can be useful for justifying further stewardship resources.

Van den Bosch and colleagues[28] sought to determine quality indicators that could be used to describe appropriate antibiotic use in patients with bacterial infections who are not in the intensive care unit. Using the RAND modified Delphi method, the group identified several quality indicators for ASP use. Obtaining cultures before initiation of antibiotics, prescribing appropriate empirical therapy based on local and national guidelines, and appropriate de-escalation and pathogen-directed therapy received the highest scores among those selected.[28] Thus, it is reasonable for ASPs to track and report compliance with these or other institutional-specific quality measures as an internal metric for appropriateness of antibiotic use.

MEASURING ECONOMIC OUTCOMES

An additional metric that is commonly measured by ASPs is antimicrobial costs. Several studies have proven that ASPs can significantly decrease costs by improving antimicrobial use, usually within the first few years of program development, after which drug costs and savings often stabilize.[5,29–31] In times of cost neutrality, it is important to emphasize to hospital administrators that costs will increase, and quality of patient care will decrease if the program is terminated.[1] The economic impact of program termination was described in a study by Standiford and colleagues[5]; after the 7-year program ended, expenses skyrocketed, strongly suggesting that the program was maintaining financial stability.

In a survey to physicians and pharmacists in acute care hospitals in the United States, hospital administrators and pharmacy directors still perceived cost as the most important outcome for ASPs, whereas infectious diseases physicians perceived patient outcomes and appropriateness of antimicrobial use as the most important metrics.[32] The culture of prioritizing decreased antimicrobial costs while at the very least not increasing harm to patients should be refocused. The underlying goal of an ASP is to improve patient care, and decreased costs should not take precedence over improved outcomes. As the reimbursement model in the US health care system has evolved from fee-for-service to that of quality of care, ASPs should shift toward outcome-driven metrics.[10] By prioritizing quality and health outcomes, ASPs can uniquely position themselves as essential players in health care reform by improving quality of care.

Because the primary goal for hospital administrators is to improve patient care *and* ensure economic vitality of the institution, demonstrating financial stability, at the very least, will likely remain a metric to be tracked and reported. When measuring costs, the 2016 IDSA/SHEA ASP Guidelines recommend that antibiotic expenditures be measured as administration data rather than purchasing data and normalized to patient census (as stated in **Table 1**).[2] Focusing on cost-effectiveness by incorporating overall health care–associated costs or savings is more valuable than antimicrobial costs alone and also should be tracked and measured when performing cost analyses.[1,10]

MEASURING CLINICAL OUTCOMES

Clinical outcome measures are more impactful than cost and process measures and are the result of improvements in quality measures; however, even some AMS experts are reluctant to routinely measure clinical outcomes.[8] The Structured Taskforce of Experts Working at Reliable Standards for Stewardship (STEWARDS) panel identified 6 appropriate metrics to assess the impact of ASP interventions (2 measures of *Clostridium difficile* infection [CDI] incidence, incidence of drug-resistant pathogens, DOT over admission, DOT over patient days, and redundant therapy events).[8] The panel members were hesitant to include additional clinical outcomes as metrics due to concerns with attributing outcomes exclusively to an ASP intervention and the need to tease out confounding factors. Appropriate clinical outcome measures are not well-defined, and more research is needed to identify optimal clinical outcome metrics for ASP purposes.[8,10,32] Outcome metrics recommended by the IDSA/SHEA ASP Guidelines and the CDC's Core Elements mirror those chosen by the STEWARDS panel and include rates of hospital-onset CDI and antibiotic resistance, although the guidelines recognize that even these metrics can be influenced by confounding factors.[1,2]

Nagel and colleagues[10] recommend that ASP personnel partner with hospital administrators to establish institutional-specific outcome measures and formulate a plan to meet specific goals. Decreasing inpatient length of hospitalization and promoting early transition to outpatient care are potential goals to set regarding all hospitalized patients or a subset of patients with specific infectious diseases. Additional outcome metrics could include mortality, mortality related to antibiotic-resistant pathogens, infection-related mortality (although there is no standardized definition), hospital readmission rates, reinfection rates, and infection-related complications.[10]

The group also believes attention should be given to those outcome metrics that hospitals are evaluated against. Because the Centers for Medicare and Medicaid Services (CMS) requires hospitals to report hospital-acquired CDI and hospital-acquired methicillin-resistant *Staphylococcus aureus* (MRSA) bloodstream infections, these infections are routinely scrutinized by hospital administrators.[33] Thus, focusing on interventions and metrics surrounding these disease states is important. Several studies have suggested that an ASP review and intervention following real-time alerts in patients with bacteremia can decrease mortality, length of hospitalization, and hospital costs.[34–38]

Other national quality indicators supported by CMS and the Joint Commission that are associated with ASP include 30-day mortality rates and 30-day readmission rates in patients with pneumonia.[39] Additionally, ASP programs can help meet the Surgical Care Improvement Program measures, which focus on appropriate timing of administration and discontinuation of preoperative antibiotics and selecting the most appropriate antibiotic to decrease surgical site infections.[40]

Although it may be challenging to solely attribute an ASP intervention to an improvement in patient outcomes, appropriate clinical outcome metrics should be further developed, validated, and standardized. More research is needed to define optimal outcome metrics, particularly for external benchmarking purposes. As many ASP interventions have resulted in an improvement in clinical outcomes, these studies could serve as a basis for programs to refocus their energy on patient outcomes.

OUTPATIENT ANTIMICROBIAL STEWARDSHIP METRICS

The urgent need to improve use of antibiotics across the patient care continuum includes the need to develop appropriate ASP metrics in the outpatient setting. More than 60% of human antibiotic use occurs in the outpatient setting, and data suggest that non–first-line regimens are selected nearly 50% of the time.[41,42] There are currently no standardized metrics for outpatient ASP. Measuring antimicrobial use stratified by prescriber, diagnosis, and antibiotic is an appropriate metric to start with. Developing antimicrobial guidelines for the most frequent diagnoses for which antibiotics are prescribed (ie, skin and soft tissue infections, respiratory tract infections, and urinary tract infections), and measuring compliance with those guidelines could help identify future targets for stewardship.[11,43,44] Additional metrics to consider for outpatient ASPs mirror many of those that are used for the inpatient setting and can be found in **Table 3**.

FUTURE CONSIDERATIONS/SUMMARY

ASPs require validated and standardized metrics to demonstrate impact. The most commonly used metrics measure antimicrobial consumption, such as DOT per 1000 days present or DOT per 1000 patient days. Consumption metrics can be submitted to the CDC's NHSN AU module for national benchmarking purposes. Historically, measuring antimicrobial costs has been important for program justification to hospital administration. ASPs should focus on more meaningful cost analyses, including total health care costs. The most commonly measured clinical outcomes include incidence of CDI and drug-resistant bacteria. Future research is needed to develop additional clinical outcome metrics and metrics for the outpatient setting. In the interim, programs should partner with hospital administrators to develop institutional-specific clinical outcome measures to improve patient care and use previous studies that have shown improvements in clinical outcomes as leverage.

Table 3	
Potential metrics for outpatient antibiotic stewardship programs	
Measures	**Metrics**
Antimicrobial consumption	Antimicrobial prescribing rates by drug, diagnosis, and prescriber
Quality/Process	Local or national guideline compliance Unnecessary prescribing for syndromes that do not require antibiotics (eg, asymptomatic bacteriuria, viral illnesses, acute bronchitis, nonsuppurative otitis media) Vaccination rates
Clinical outcomes	Clinical and microbiologic cure Treatment failure Rate of CA-CDI Rate of drug-resistant pathogens
Unintended consequences	Adverse drug events/toxicities Rates of hospital admission, emergency department visits, or return office visits

Abbreviations: CA, community acquired; CDI, *Clostridium difficile* infection.
Data from Refs.[11,43,44]

REFERENCES

1. Pollack LA, Srinivasan A. Core elements of hospital antibiotic stewardship programs from the Centers for Disease Control and Prevention. Clin Infect Dis 2014;59(Suppl 3):S97–100.
2. Barlam TF, Cosgrove SE, Abbo LM, et al. Implementing an antibiotic stewardship program: guidelines by the Infectious Diseases Society of America and the Society for Healthcare Epidemiology of America. Clin Infect Dis 2016;62(10):e51–77.
3. Goff DA, Bauer KA, Reed EE, et al. Is the "low-hanging fruit" worth picking for antimicrobial stewardship programs? Clin Infect Dis 2012;55(4):587–92.
4. MacDougall C, Polk RE. Antimicrobial stewardship programs in health care systems. Clin Microbiol Rev 2005;18(4):638–56.
5. Standiford HC, Chan S, Tripoli M, et al. Antimicrobial stewardship at a large tertiary care academic medical center: cost analysis before, during, and after a 7-year program. Infect Control Hosp Epidemiol 2012;33(4):338–45.
6. Ibrahim OM, Polk RE. Antimicrobial use metrics and benchmarking to improve stewardship outcomes: methodology, opportunities, and challenges. Infect Dis Clin North Am 2014;28(2):195–214.
7. Shlaes DM, Gerding DN, John JF Jr, et al. Society for Healthcare Epidemiology of America and Infectious Diseases Society of America joint committee on the prevention of antimicrobial resistance: guidelines for the prevention of antimicrobial resistance in hospitals. Clin Infect Dis 1997;25(3):584–99.
8. Moehring RW, Anderson DJ, Cochran RL, et al. Expert consensus on metrics to assess the impact of patient-level antimicrobial stewardship interventions in acute-care settings. Clin Infect Dis 2017;64(3):377–83.
9. Society for Healthcare Epidemiology of America, Infectious Diseases Society of America, Peadiatric Infectious Diseases Society. Policy statement on antimicrobial stewardship by the Society for Healthcare Epidemiology of America (SHEA), the Infectious Diseases Society of America (IDSA), and the Pediatric Infectious Diseases Society (PIDS). Infect Control Hosp Epidemiol 2012;33(4):322–7.
10. Nagel JL, Stevenson JG, Eiland EH 3rd, et al. Demonstrating the value of antimicrobial stewardship programs to hospital administrators. Clin Infect Dis 2014;59(Suppl 3):S146–53.
11. Sanchez GV, Fleming-Dutra KE, Roberts RM, et al. Core elements of outpatient antibiotic stewardship. MMWR Recomm Rep 2016;65(6):1–12.
12. The White House. National Action Plan for Combating Antibiotic-Resistant Bacteria. Available at: https://obamawhitehouse.archives.gov/sites/default/files/docs/national_action_plan_for_combating_antibotic-resistant_bacteria.pdf. Accessed April 22, 2018.
13. Dellit TH, Owens RC, McGowan JE Jr, et al. Infectious Diseases Society of America and the Society for Healthcare Epidemiology of America guidelines for developing an institutional program to enhance antimicrobial stewardship. Clin Infect Dis 2007;44(2):159–77.
14. Scheckler WE, Bennett JV. Antibiotic use in seven community hospitals. JAMA 1970;213:264–7.
15. Shapiro M, Townsend TR, Rosner B, et al. Use of antimicrobial drugs in general hospitals. II. Analysis of patterns of use. J Infect Dis 1979;139:698–706.
16. Craig WA, Uman SJ, Shaw WR, et al. Hospital use of antimicrobial drugs. Survey at 19 hospitals and results of antimicrobial control program. Ann Intern Med 1978;89(5 Pt 2 Suppl):793–5.

17. Polk RE, Fox C, Mahoney A, et al. Measurement of adult antibacterial drug use in 130 US hospitals: comparison of defined daily dose and days of therapy. Clin Infect Dis 2007;44(5):664–70.

18. Moehring RW, Dodds Ashley ES, Ren X, et al. Denominator matters in estimating antimicrobial use: a comparison of days present and patient days. Infect Control Hosp Epidemiol 2018;39(5):612–5.

19. WHO Collaborating Centre for Drug Statistics Methodology, Guidelines for ATC classification and DDD assignment 2018. Oslo (Norway): 2017.

20. Morris AM. Antimicrobial stewardship programs: appropriate measures and metrics to study their impact. Curr Treat Options Infect Dis 2014;6(2):101–12.

21. Zagorski BM, Trick WE, Schwartz DN, et al. The effect of renal dysfunction on antimicrobial use measurements. Clin Infect Dis 2002;35(12):1491–7.

22. Kullar R, Goff DA, Schulz LT, et al. The "epic" challenge of optimizing antimicrobial stewardship: the role of electronic medical records and technology. Clin Infect Dis 2013;57(7):1005–13.

23. Centers for Disease Control and Prevention. Antimicrobial use and resistance (AUR) module. Available at: http://www.cdc.gov/nhsn//pscManual/pscAURcurrent.pdf. Accessed April 12, 2018.

24. Mandy B, Koutny E, Cornette C, et al. Methodological validation of monitoring indicators of antibiotics use in hospitals. Pharm World Sci 2004;26(2):90–5.

25. Momattin H, Al-Ali AY, Mohammed K, et al. Benchmarking of antibiotic usage: an adjustment to reflect antibiotic stewardship program outcome in a hospital in Saudi Arabia. J Infect Public Health 2017. https://doi.org/10.1016/j.jiph.2017.08.008.

26. Dalton BR, Sabuda DM, Bresee LC, et al. Assessment of antimicrobial utilization metrics: days of therapy versus defined daily doses and pharmacy dispensing records versus nursing administration data. Infect Control Hosp Epidemiol 2015;36(6):688–94.

27. Bennett N, Schulz L, Boyd S, et al. Understanding inpatient antimicrobial stewardship metrics. Am J Health Syst Pharm 2018;75(4):230–8.

28. van den Bosch CM, Geerlings SE, Natsch S, et al. Quality indicators to measure appropriate antibiotic use in hospitalized adults. Clin Infect Dis 2015;60(2):281–91.

29. Nowak MA, Nelson RE, Breidenbach JL, et al. Clinical and economic outcomes of a prospective antimicrobial stewardship program. Am J Health Syst Pharm 2012;69(17):1500–8.

30. Beardsley JR, Williamson JC, Johnson JW, et al. Show me the money: long-term financial impact of an antimicrobial stewardship program. Infect Control Hosp Epidemiol 2012;33(4):398–400.

31. Agwu AL, Lee CK, Jain SK, et al. A World Wide Web-based antimicrobial stewardship program improves efficiency, communication, and user satisfaction and reduces cost in a tertiary care pediatric medical center. Clin Infect Dis 2008;47(6):747–53.

32. Bumpass JB, McDaneld PM, DePestel DD, et al. Outcomes and metrics for antimicrobial stewardship: survey of physicians and pharmacists. Clin Infect Dis 2014;59(Suppl 3):S108–11.

33. Centers for Medicare and Medicaid Services. Hospital-Acquired Condition (HAC) Reduction Program. Available at: https://www.cms.gov/Medicare/Quality-Initiatives-Patient-Assessment-Instruments/Value-Based-Programs/HAC/Hospital-Acquired-Conditions.html. Accessed April 12, 2018.

34. Pogue JM, Mynatt RP, Marchaim D, et al. Automated alerts coupled with antimicrobial stewardship intervention lead to decreases in length of stay in patients with gram-negative bacteremia. Infect Control Hosp Epidemiol 2014;35(2):132–8.

35. Huang AM, Newton D, Kunapuli A, et al. Impact of rapid organism identification via matrix-assisted laser desorption/ionization time-of-flight combined with antimicrobial stewardship team intervention in adult patients with bacteremia and candidemia. Clin Infect Dis 2013;57(9):1237–45.

36. Goff DA, Jankowski C, Tenover FC. Using rapid diagnostic tests to optimize antimicrobial selection in antimicrobial stewardship programs. Pharmacotherapy 2012;32(8):677–87.

37. Muto CA, Blank MK, Marsh JW, et al. Control of an outbreak of infection with the hypervirulent *Clostridium difficile* BI strain in a university hospital using a comprehensive "bundle" approach. Clin Infect Dis 2007;45(10):1266–73.

38. Valiquette L, Cossette B, Garant MP, et al. Impact of a reduction in the use of high-risk antibiotics on the course of an epidemic of *Clostridium difficile*-associated disease caused by the hypervirulent NAP1/027 strain. Clin Infect Dis 2007;45(Suppl 2):S112–21.

39. The Joint Commission. Specifications manual for national hospital inpatient quality measures. Available at: http://www.jointcommission.org/specifications_manual_for_national_hospital_inpatient_quality_measures.aspx. Accessed April 14, 2018.

40. Institute for Healthcare Improvement. Surgical care improvement project. Available at: http://www.ihi.org/resources/Pages/OtherWebsites/SurgicalCare ImprovementProject.aspx. Accessed April 20, 2018.

41. Suda KJ, Hicks LA, Roberts RM, et al. A national evaluation of antibiotic expenditures by healthcare setting in the United States, 2009. J Antimicrob Chemother 2013;68(3):715–8.

42. Hersh AL, Fleming-Dutra KE, Shapiro DJ, et al, Outpatient Antibiotic Use Target-Setting Workgroup. Frequency of first-line antibiotic selection among US ambulatory care visits for otitis media, sinusitis, and pharyngitis. JAMA Intern Med 2016; 176(12):1870–2.

43. Klepser ME, Dobson EL, Pogue JM, et al. A call to action for outpatient antibiotic stewardship. J Am Pharm Assoc (2003) 2017;57(4):457–63.

44. Dobson EL, Klepser ME, Pogue JM, et al. Outpatient antibiotic stewardship: interventions and opportunities. J Am Pharm Assoc (2003) 2017;57(4):464–73.

Moving?

Make sure your subscription moves with you!

To notify us of your new address, find your **Clinics Account Number** (located on your mailing label above your name), and contact customer service at:

Email: journalscustomerservice-usa@elsevier.com

800-654-2452 (subscribers in the U.S. & Canada)
314-447-8871 (subscribers outside of the U.S. & Canada)

Fax number: 314-447-8029

Elsevier Health Sciences Division
Subscription Customer Service
3251 Riverport Lane
Maryland Heights, MO 63043

*To ensure uninterrupted delivery of your subscription, please notify us at least 4 weeks in advance of move.

Printed and bound by CPI Group (UK) Ltd, Croydon, CR0 4YY

03/10/2024

01040849-0008